Danelina Vacheva

Rehabilitation and occupational therapy in some common motor deficits

Danelina Vacheva

Rehabilitation and occupational therapy in some common motor deficits

LAP LAMBERT Academic Publishing

Impressum / Imprint

Bibliografische Information der Deutschen Nationalbibliothek: Die Deutsche Nationalbibliothek verzeichnet diese Publikation in der Deutschen Nationalbibliografie; detaillierte bibliografische Daten sind im Internet über http://dnb.d-nb.de abrufbar.

Alle in diesem Buch genannten Marken und Produktnamen unterliegen warenzeichen-, marken- oder patentrechtlichem Schutz bzw. sind Warenzeichen oder eingetragene Warenzeichen der jeweiligen Inhaber. Die Wiedergabe von Marken, Produktnamen, Gebrauchsnamen, Handelsnamen, Warenbezeichnungen u.s.w. in diesem Werk berechtigt auch ohne besondere Kennzeichnung nicht zu der Annahme, dass solche Namen im Sinne der Warenzeichen- und Markenschutzgesetzgebung als frei zu betrachten wären und daher von jedermann benutzt werden dürften.

Bibliographic information published by the Deutsche Nationalbibliothek: The Deutsche Nationalbibliothek lists this publication in the Deutsche Nationalbibliografie; detailed bibliographic data are available in the Internet at http://dnb.d-nb.de.

Any brand names and product names mentioned in this book are subject to trademark, brand or patent protection and are trademarks or registered trademarks of their respective holders. The use of brand names, product names, common names, trade names, product descriptions etc. even without a particular marking in this works is in no way to be construed to mean that such names may be regarded as unrestricted in respect of trademark and brand protection legislation and could thus be used by anyone.

Coverbild / Cover image: www.ingimage.com

Verlag / Publisher:
LAP LAMBERT Academic Publishing
ist ein Imprint der / is a trademark of
AV Akademikerverlag GmbH & Co. KG
Heinrich-Böcking-Str. 6-8, 66121 Saarbrücken, Deutschland / Germany
Email: info@lap-publishing.com

Herstellung: siehe letzte Seite /
Printed at: see last page
ISBN: 978-3-659-45076-1

Copyright © 2013 AV Akademikerverlag GmbH & Co. KG
Alle Rechte vorbehalten. / All rights reserved. Saarbrücken 2013

CONTENTS

Introduction	6
The Place of Occupational Therapy in Medical Rehabilitation	7
The Role of the Thumb for the Function of the Hand	9
Anatomical Characteristics of the Hand	10
Functional Characteristic of the Hand	13
Test for Comprehensive Functional Assessment of Radioulnar Joints, Wrist Joints and Fingers	16
Occupational therapy in traumas of the hand	18
Complex Program in Physiotherapy and Rehabilitation	19
Test for activities of daily living	20
Medical Rehabilitation and Occupational Therapy after Mamestomiya	23
Program in Kinesitherapy	24
Test Activities of Daily Living (toilet and personal hygiene)	26
Medical Rehabilitation and Occupational Therapy in Patients with Lesion of Plexus Brachialis	28
Anatomy, Etiology and Pathogenesis	28
Diagnosis and Treatment	30
Complex Program in Physiotherapy and Rehabilitation	31
Results from a Clinical Study of Patients with Plexopathy of Plexus Brachialis	32
Occupational Therapy in Patients who suffer from Cerebral Vascular Disease	38
Results from a Clinical Study in Patients suffering from Cerebral Vascular Disease	39
Test Activities of Daily Living (activities for preparing food and feeding)	40
Test Activities of Daily Living (toilet and personal hygiene)	43
Medical Rehabilitation and Occupational Therapy among Patients with Arthroplastic Hip Joint	50
Program in Kinesitherapy and Training Walking Assistive Devices	51
Conclusion	53
References	54

COMMONLY USED ABBREVIATIONS

Activities of Daily Living	ADL
Dominant limb	DL
Not- dominant limb	NDL

Introduction

It is a common knowledge that rehabilitation is practicing all means that pursue reduced levels of incapacity to work and disability, and training people with permanent incapacity to reach optimum social integration. The rehabilitation is a complex of joint, coordinated medical, social, pedagogical and professional actions, for persons with reduced capacity to work (due to disease or other injury), in order to achieve the maximum possible physical, psychic and labor fitness. The major divisions are medical and psychological, occupational and professional, and social and legal rehabilitation. According to modern understanding, the rehabilitation is a *functional therapy*, based on precise *functional assessment.*

During all stages of the recovery process, the main **tasks** are: monitoring of the effect of applied complex treatment and rehabilitation, and assessment of rehabilitation potential; ensuring the quality of life of patients through timely, competent and suitable selection of physical means and methods; participation in drawing up medical appraisal report, for solving professional and social problems of persons in danger of disability.

The physical and rehabilitation medicine applies bio-psycho-social model of disability, based on the International Classification of Functioning, Disability and Health, developed by the World Health Organization.

The right to have access to rehabilitation after health damage or disease is a basic human right. The specialists in medical rehabilitation and ergotherapy are tutors of the patient with temporary or permanent incapacity to work, due to health damage or disease. The final target of this training is acquiring skills, needed in patient's everyday life, i.e. *"how to do"* and *"how to perform a task"* instructions.

THE PLACE OF OCCUPATIONAL THERAPY IN MEDICAL REHABILITATION

The dynamic life of people, multiplied traumatism, unceasing industrial failures, natural calamities and military confrontations lead to increased sick rate of muscle and skeleton system diseases worldwide. We encounter more often problems of individuals in active age, with permanent neuromuscular and psychological disabilities, which must have assistant in their daily life.[1]

This requires complex rehabilitation and socio-economic life of people with disabilities to support. It is imperative to adjust the household environment to motor features of the individual.[2, 3] With these issues are being addressed occupational therapy. Occupational therapy professionals have knowledge of the fundamental sciences: Anatomy, Physiology, Kinesiology, methods and tests for functional evaluation of organs and systems, as well as their pathology sections; major clinic disciplines as Orthopedics and Traumatology, Neurology, Pediatrics, Internal Diseases, Surgery Diseases, Kinesiotherapy, manual techniques, pre-formed physical factors, ergotherapeutical and pedagogical methods of work.[4]

Accumulated fundamental knowledge is supplemented with ergonomy, prosthesis and use of orthesis, auxiliary aid for movement (crutches, cane, support chair, wheelchair), equipment and devices, facilitating the everyday life of people

---

[1] Koleva I. Capabilities of modern physical and rehabilitation medicine to improve the quality of life patients. Rehabilitation medicine and quality of life. 2007; 1(1):4-13 [In Bulgarian].
[2] Kaplan E, Tzurengapova D, Shantanova L. Optimization of the adaptive processes of the organism. – Moskow: Science. 1990; 137-149.
[3] Kielhofner GA. Model of Human Occupation. – Baltimore: Williams & Wilkins. 1995; 80-93.
[4] Ministry of Education, Bulgaria. Ordinance on Unified State Requirements for Obtaining Higher Education in professional field of "Health Care" educational and qualification degree "specialist". Published by the Official Gazette, number 95/ 29.11.2005 [In Bulgarian].

with disabilities –toilet and hygiene needs, dressing and putting shoes on, cooking and eating, various domestic and occupational activities.[1]

The whole training of such type of specialists requires a serious fundamental theoretical background and significant practical training.[2] The curriculum includes lectures, seminars and clinical practice for trainees conducted at the University Hospital in Pleven.[3] The lecture course is delivered by habilitated lecturers in scientific disciplines; the seminars are conducted by assistant lecturers and chief assistant lecturers of corresponding departments and the practical training in special subjects is completed as procedures in kinesitherapy and healing massage by the students.[4]

The clinical practice is connected with immediate work with patients (fig. 1) and severely injured individuals, who later live with these injuries and are called clients of health care.

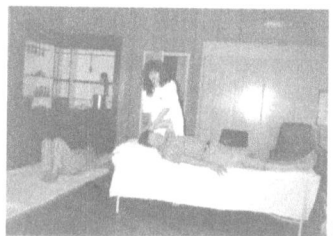 Fig. 1 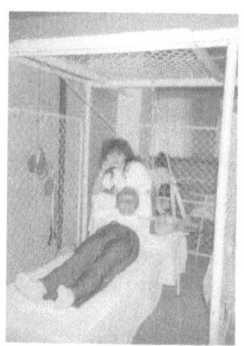 Fig. 2

For the construction and improvement of occupational therapy professionals considerable importance there is the practical training and proper mastering of

---

[1] Koleva I. Professional competence of bachelors in Medical Rehabilitation and Ergotherapy, as members of the rehabilitation team. Prevention and rehabilitation. 2008; 2(1): 2-7 [In Bulgaria].
[2] Nabi A. The innovative work of the teacher in the system of quality assurance. Problms of modern Philology, Pedagogics and Pshichology. Materials digest of the XXV International Scientific and Practical Conference in Pedagogics, Pshichological sciences and the Philological sciences. Pedagogical Sciences. – London. 2012; 17-19 [In Russian].
[3] Ministry of Health – Programme Phare. Health reform in Bulgaria. Collection of lectures, first part. Floor. order. Prof. M. Popov. – Sofia: Makedonia press. 1997; 382 [In Bulgarian].
[4] Petkova I. Interactive methods in the qualification of professionals working in institutions. Collection of materials International cientific conferention "Interactive methods in modern education" West University „Neofit Rilski". – Blagoevgrad: Sani – H and H OOD. 2010; 368-373 [In Bulgarian].

various methods and manual therapeutic techniques, like manual traction and mobilization of peripheral joints, neuro-muscular facilitation, post-isometric relaxation of shortened muscles, the muscle test method, sling suspension (fig. 2) and pull therapy.[1]

The time of rapid developments we live in, Bulgaria's membership in the European Union and imposed changes and requirements to our public health system necessitated to educate and train specialists in Medical Rehabilitation and Ergotherapy, who can provide early rehabilitation at paramedical and medical institutions, sanatoria and balneology centres, various social institutions and daycare centres and dispensary for people with disabilities –children (fig. 3, 4) and adults.[2]

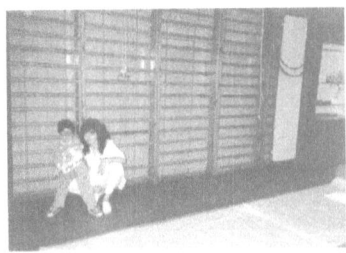
Fig. 3

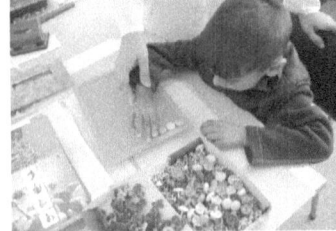
Fig. 4

The ergotherapy deals with everyday health and social issues of people with motive system damages, their self-service and daily routine.

ROLE OF POLLEX FOR HAND FUNCTION

The hand is able to perform all the complex and multilateral activities, thanks to the rare qualities that possess: high sensitivity, rich motor capabilities with significant clamping force and enviable coordination and finesse, realize on the basis of perfect cyber regulation.[3]

---

[1] Hamonet CL, Heuleu JN. Rééducation fonctionnelle et réadaptation. – Paris – New York – Barcelona – Milan: Masson. 1998; 164-168.
[2] AOTA Council on Standards. Occupational therapy – its definition and function. Amer. J. Occup. Therapy. 1972; (26): 204-205.
[3] Bosnev V, Matev I. Disease of the hand. – Sofia: Medicine and Physical Culture. 1989; 174-175 [In Bulgarian].

Anatomical Characteristics of the Hand

Skeleton hand – **manus** – consists of three located one after the other groups of bones [1] : ossa carpi (fig. 5), ossa metacarpalia and phalanges (fig. 6).

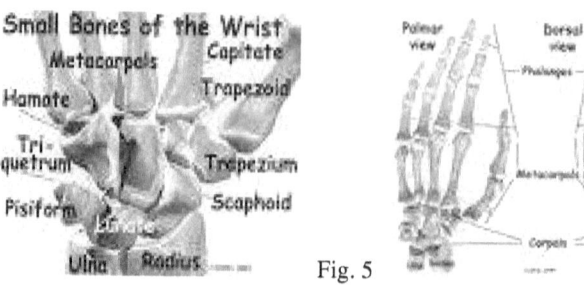

Fig. 5   Fig. 6

The bones of the fingers (phalanges) are primary, secondary and nail. The pollex has only basic and nail phalanx.

The bones of the hand (**manus**) are combined together into two groups joints: joints of the wrist and joints of the fingers. In *art. carpometacarpea* of fingers II-V movements are insignificant and have springy characteristic, while *art. carpometacarpea pollicis* is completely independent. In it are combined trapezoidal bone at the base of the first metacarpalia bone (fig. 6). Articular surfaces are saddle-shaped, which allows two degrees freedom of movement on two main axes: on the front-rear axis is carried abduction and adduction 45-60° and a transverse axis – flexion and opponents of pollex to the other fingers and extension – reset total 35-40°. The looseness of this joint allows rotation around the longitudinal axis, which favors the opposition of the thumb and increases immensely gripping capabilities of hand. *Articulatio metacarpophalangeal pollicis* is cumulus and has three degrees freedom of movement: movements in the sagittal plane from 30-90° flexion and 5-10°

---

[1] Sinelnikov R. Atlas of Human Anatomy. – Moskow: Medicine. 1978; 261-272 [In Russian].

extension.[1] Details of movements in the frontal plane is occur rarely in the literature – about 30° abduction and 10° adduction.[2]

In *Articulationes interphalangeae* takes placearticulation between the phalanges of the fingers like pollex have only one joint and it can be done flexion about 90°.

Bones, joints and skeletal muscles build motor apparatus of the human. Bones and joints compose passive part of motor aparatus, while muscles compose its active part, because the movements are the result of their cuts.

Antebrachial muscles acting on the pollex: ***m. flexor pollicis longus*** flexes the pollex in all his joints and participate in manus adduction (n. medianus); ***m. abductor pollicis longus*** makes abduction os metacarpi pollicis and of hand in wrist (n. radialis); ***m. extensor pollicis brevis*** in wrist and metacarpi joint pollicis support abduction, and essentially extends the main phalanx of pollex (n. radialis); ***m. extensor pollicis longus*** extends the pollex in all his joints and of hand in wrist (n. radialis).[3]

The muscles of pollex are small, short, four in number, forming the cushion of the pollex – *thenar*: ***m. abductor pollicis brevis*** abduct ossa metacarpalia of the pollex and extends the pollex in the main phalanx (n. medianus); ***m. flexor pollicis brevis*** flexes the pollex and supporting its opposition to the other fingers (n. medianus); ***m. opponens pollicis*** oppose the pollex to the other fingers (n. medianus); ***m. adductor pollicis*** flexes the main phalanx and adduct the pollex thus supports the opposition of the pollex to the other fingers (n. ulnaris).[4]

---

[1] Regan WD, Korinek SL, Morrey BF ann KN. Biomechanical Study of igaments around the Elbow Joint. Clin. Orthop. 1991; 170-179.
[2] Kalchev I, Morova E. Kinesiology. – Sofia: University "Sv. Kliment Ohridski". 1993; 45-52 [In Bulgarian].
[3] Morov Sp. Human Anatomy. – Sofia: Medicine and Physical Culture. 1981; 68-91[In Bulgarian].
[4] Kojuharov V. Kinesiology analysis of the gripping power of the hand with fingers reconstructed. Proceedings of II Congress of the Association of Kinesitherapeutists Rehabilitators and Bulgaria. Sofia, 1989; 13-15 [In Bulgarian].

Great mobility, autonomy and diversity of the movements of the thumb due to the fact that these small muscles always act synchronously with its larger muscles located in the forearm.[1]

The muscles of the hand made fine, small, coordinating movements, which they complement the activity of the muscles and give predmishnichnite hand dexterity, accuracy and precision grip, so necessary for employment rights.[2]

Wrist forms a flexible connection between the forearm and hand, and it have kinesiologic task is to optimally positioned to perform fine motor actions.

Many good coordination in the operation of various motor elements is carried out by the coordination of muscle activity – involving several muscle and each performs different tasks: as *agonists, antagonists, stabilizers and neutralizers*.[3]

Significant mobility in each of the individual elements *(rays)* is due to the large number of contained therein kinetic couples (joints), and large number of muscles with diverse and highly differentiated action securing fine and precise movements of each element of the kinetic chain.

The role of the **pollex** of the hand is determined by the fact that only there have independent **articulatio carpo-metacarpea**, which made complex movement (begins with abduction, passing in adduction and slight flexion in metakarpophalangeal and interphalangeal joints, ends with rotation and opposition). This allows him to perform opposing the other fingers *(opposition)* and making **hookup** – function of the human hand is brought to perfection.[4]

Figure 7 presents fingers shaped like a butterfly with a rigid body and flexible wings. Position of "wings" helps the opposition of pollex to the little finger. Radial "wing" is more mobile and shorter than the ulnar due to the mobility of the first carpo-metacarpal joint of pollex.

---

[1] Matev I. Reconstructive surgery of the thumb. – Sofia: Medicine and Physical Culture. 1978, 14-25. In Bulgarian].

[2] Kaptelin LF, Lasskay LA. Occupational therapy in traumatology and orthopedics. – Moscow: Medicine. 1979; 91-93[In Russian].

[3] Kapandji IA. The physiology of the joints. – London: Livingstone. 1970; 72-79.

[4] Matev I, Bankov St. Rehabilitation of Hand Inguries. – Sofia: Medicine and Physical Culture. 1977; 32-38 [In Bulgarian].

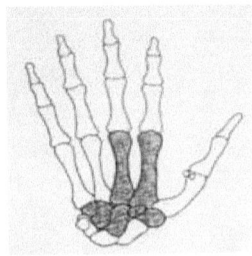 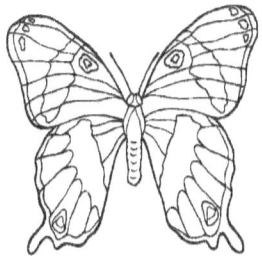

Fig .7   Scheme of mobile and fixed structure of hand

If damage or loss of pollex (amputation), the hand loses over 70% of working capacity, especially if the affected dominant upper limb.

Functional Characteristic of the Hand

Along with goniometry applied to measure the larger joints are used and some tests to determine the mobility of the fingers. These are the different types of prehensile movements (grip – the hand ability to cover and hold different objects).[1]

The movements of the hand (wrist and fingers) are two main groups (fig. 8):

* ***Non prehensile movements*** – the object is influenced by pushing, clapping, lifting movements of the hand or fingers separated;

* ***Prehensile movements (grips)*** – the object wholly or partly can cover and hold with the palm and fingers, in which participate all joints of the hand simultaneously. In view of the position of the hand and its function the grips are power *(spherical, cylindrical, fist, as hook)* and precision *(peak, palmar, scissor, as key)*.

---

[1] Matev I, Bankov St. Rehabilitation of Hand Inguries. – Sofia: Medicine and Physical Culture. 1977; 79-84 [In Bulgarian].

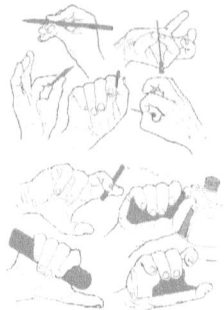

Fig. 8   Types of grips (precision and power)

In the **power grip** (fig. 9, 10) the object is squeezed between part of the fingers flexion and palm, as the thumb and thenar are the mainstay of the hand which opposing the pressure of fingers and contributes to grip strength.

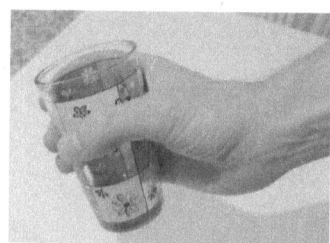 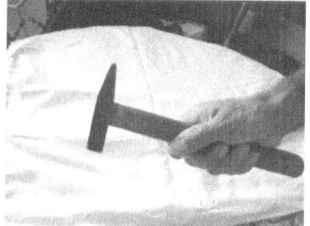

Fig. 9   Fig. 10

In **precision grip** – pulps of the pollex and forefinger withstand and perform sophisticated actions of the hand (fig. 11, 12).

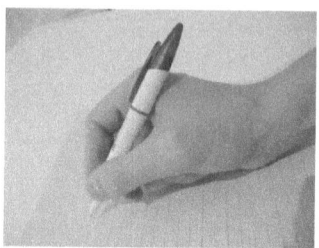 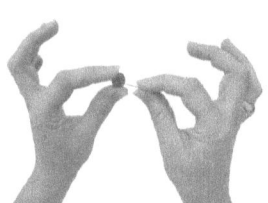

Fig. 11   Fig. 12

When necessary grip with maximum force, **functional position of the wrist** is the extension (20-35°) and light ulnar deviation (10-15°). When necessary grip with maximum force, functional position of the wrist is extension and light ulnar deviation. This position allows full flexion of the fingers as the wrist extensors stabilize grip. In flexion of the wrist grip strength decreased significantly. The reasons for this are that the flexors of the fingers go into active disease and extensors in a passive failure (fig.13).[1]

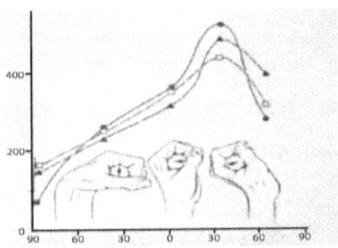

Fig. 13   Position of the wrist determining grip strength

For work hands in daily life is characterized by constant, but varied physical activity. Perform more movements and less maintaining certain static positions.

Many coordination in the operation of various engine components gives great practical possibilities for complex and precise movements combined, both volume and degree of freedom of movement, and coordination of muscular activity.

Kinetic analysis of hand movements and technological analysis of the different work activities are reliable tool for selecting the most appropriate work activities and daily living activities, contributing to a better functional recovery of traumatized limb.[2]

---

[1] Karaneshev G, Milcheva D. Methods for diagnostics and examination in remedial gymnastics. – Sofia: National Sport Academy. 1984; 26-73 [In Bulgarian].
[2] Kaptelin LF, Lasskay LA. Occupational therapy in traumatology and orthopedics. – Moscow: Medicine. 1979; 131-132 [In Russian].

Test for Comprehensive Functional Assessment of Radioulnar Joints, Wrist joints and Fingers

Similar to the test UCLA (C. Rockwood, F. Matsen, 1998)[1] to functional assessment of the shoulder joint and test W. D. Regan (1991)[2] to functional assessment of the elbow and radioulnar joints, modified by N. Popov (2003), we offer specially designed by our test to research and reporting of **comprehensive functional status**[3], of patiens after trauma and diseases of the upper limb – radioulnar joints, wrist joints and fingers.

TEST
for Comprehensive Functional Assessment of Radioulnar Joints,
Wrist Joints and Fingers

№	Type of test	Test – points	Before	After	Difference
1.	Pain – 20 p.	0 p. – Strong / 20 p. – Lacking			
2.	Range of movement	Total – 20 p.			
	Radioulnar Joints	Supinatio – max. 3 p. (1° = 0,03 p.)			
	max. 6 p.	Pronatio – max. 3 p. (1° = 0,03 p.)			
	Wrist Joints	Extensio – max. 3 p. (1° = 0,04 p.)			
	max. 10 p.	Flexio – max. 3 p. (1° = 0,04 p.)			
		Rad. abd. – max. 2 p. (1° = 0,08 p.)			
		Uln. add. – max. 2 p. (1° = 0,04 p.)			
	CMC joint of the pollex	Extensio – max. 1 p.			
	max. 4 p.	Flexio – max. 1 p. (1° = 0,02 p.)			
		Abd. – max. 1 p. (1° = 0,01 p.)			
		Add. – max. 1 p. (1° = 0,06 p.)			
3.	Manual Muscle Testing	Total – 14 p.			
	Radio-ulnar Joint – max. 4 p.	Supinatio – max. 2 p. (1 gr. = 0,04 p.)			
		Pronatio – max. 2 p. (1gr. = 0,04 p.)			

---

[1] Rockwood and Masten. The Shoulder. – Philadelphia: W.B. Saunders Company, 1998, 2 ed. 1316-1323.
[2] Regan WD, Korinek SL, Morrey BF ann KN. Biomechanical Study of igaments around the Elbow Joint. Clin. Orthop. 1991; 170-179.
[3] Vacheva D, Mircheva A. Complex functional assessment of recovery for injuries and diseases of the upper limb. International Scientific Conference "Modern methods and technologies in research" – Proceedings of the University of Economics – Varna. 2012; 420-462.

	Wrist Joints – **max. 6 p.**	Extensio – max. 2 p. (1 gr. = 0,04 p.)			
		Flexio – max. 2 p. (1 gr. = 0,04 p.)			
		Rad. abd. – max. 1 p. (1 gr. = 0,02 p.)			
		Uln. add. – max. 1 p. (1 gr. = 0,02 p.)			
	CMC joint of the pollex – **max. 4 p.**	Extensio – max. 1 p. (1 gr. = 0,02 p.)			
		Flexio – max. 1 p. (1 gr. = 0,02 p.)			
		Abd. – max. 1 p. (1 gr. = 0,02 p.)			
		Add. – max. 1 p. (1 gr. = 0,02 p.)			
4.	**Tests grabs**	**Total – 19 p.**			
	max. 2 p.	Spherical – (1 gr. = 0,04 p.)			
	max. 2 p.	Cylindrical – (1gr. =0,04p.)			
	max. 3 p.	Fist – (1 gr. = 0,06 p.)			
	max. 1 p.	As hook – (1 gr. = 0,02 p.)			
	max. 4 p.	Precision – (1 gr. = 0,08 p.)			
	max. 3 p.	Palmar – (1 gr. = 0,06 p.)			
	max. 3 p.	As key – (1 gr. = 0,06 p.)			
	max. 1 p.	Scissor – (1 gr. = 0,02 p.)			
5.	**ADL**	**Totalo – 27 p.**			
	max. 6 p.	Toilet and personal hygiene – (1act. = 0,7 p.)			
	max. 6 p.	Putting on shoes and clothes – (1act. = 0,5 p.)			
	max. 7 p.	Preparing food and feeding – (1act. = 0,6 p.)			
	max. 8 p.	Daily and labour activities – (1 act. = 0,6 p.)			
	Total–max100 p.				
	Index	85 – 100 p. – Excellent, 70 – 85 p. – Very good, 40 – 70 p. – Cood, Less than 40 p. – Satisfactory			

The maximum score is 100 – „Excellent" functional recovery.

The entire test consists of **five tabs:**

- Pain assessment;
- Range of movement of joints radioulnar, wrist joint, fingers and thumb;
- Muscle testing of pronation and supination in radioulnarna it, flexion and extension at the wrist joint, muscles of the fingers and thumb;
- Tests studied grabs;

- Activities of Daily Living (**ADL**) with four different parts: toilet and personal hygiene; preparing food and feeding; activities connected to putting on shoes and clothes, daily and labour activities.

Fullest possible recovery of hand requires not only recovery of individual functional parameters and the other restore the whole person of the patient's psyche, disability, social and economic status.[1]

OCCUPATIONAL THERAPY IN TRAUMAS OF THE HAND

Distal radius fracture is a common trauma, approximately 15% of all fractures among elderly people (fig 14, 15).[2]

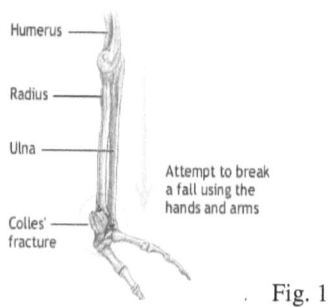

Fig. 14

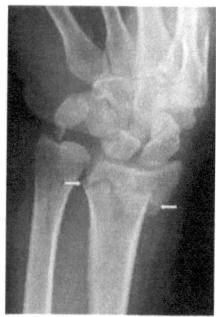

Fig. 15

In case of traumatic wrist injury one loses first their ability for self-service, they become dependent on other people's help and last but not least, they lose their labour efficiency for a certain period of time.[3,4]

The treatment of distal radius fracture is conservative – placement of plaster immobilization for 30-40 days after manual reposition [5,1,2] or operatively – by means of needles, plates, hobs or external fixture (fig. 16, 17).[3]

---

[1] Koleva I. Physical analgesia in neurological diseases. Cephalgia. 2006; 8(1):10-21 [In Bulgarian].
[2] Solgard S, Petersen VS. Epidemiology of distal radius fractures. Acta Orthop Scand. 1985; (56):391-393.
[3] Swanson AB, Matev I, G. de Groot. The strength of the hand. Bulletin of Prosthetics Research. 1970; 145-153.
[4] Topuzov I. Occupational Therapy. – Sofia: RIK Simel. II part, 2008; 101-109 [In Bulgarian].
[5] Matev I, Bankov St. Rehabilitation of Hand Inguries. – Sofia: Medicine and Physical Culture. 1977; 67-75 [In Bulgarian].

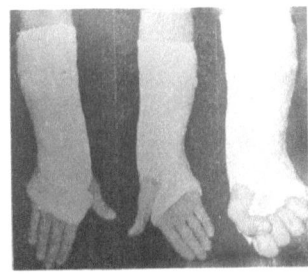 Fig. 16 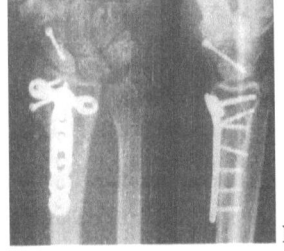 Fig. 17

After the immobilization has been removed the patients are sent for rehabilitation at the specialized departments for physical and rehabilitation medicine.[4]

Complex Program in Physiotherapy and Rehabilitation

The complex physiotherapeutic and rehabilitation program includes: ***Sub water gymnastics*** – local bath tub with water temperature 34-36° C, in the area of wrist joint and forearm (fig. 18), ***Kinesitherapy***[5] (fig. 19), ***Occupational therapy*** (fig. 20, 21), ***Impulse magnetic field*** – 15–20 min, 2 A, 1 – 100 Hz (fig. 22),, ***Interference currents*** – 5 min, 90 – 100 Hz ; 10 min 1 – 100 Hz (fig. 23), 10 procedures daily.[6, 7]

---

[1] Takov E, Tivchev P, Ivanov V. The fractures – diagnostic and treatment. – Sofia: Venel. II part, 1996; 127-135 [In Bulgarian].
[2] Yates DW. Trauma – British medical bulletin. 1999; 55(4):181-186.
[3] Alexander A.H. Bilateral traumatic dislokation of the distal radioulnar joint, ulna dorsal. – B: Case report and review of the literature. Clin Orthop. 1977; 129-238.
[4] Orjeshkovskiy VV, Volkov ES, Gabrikov NA et all. Klinicheskaya physiotherapy. – Kiev: Health. 1984; 393-395 [In Bulgarian].
[5] Slanchev P, Bonev L, Bankov St. Textbook on Kinesitherapy. – Sofia: Medicine and Physical Culture. 1986; 25-52 [In Bulgarian].
[6] Kostadinov D, Gacheva Y, Tsvetanova L. Manual Physical Therapy. – Sofia: Medicine and Physical Culture. Tom 1, 1989; 64-67 [In Bulgerian].
[7] Matev I, Bankov St. Rehabilitation of Hand Inguries. – Sofia: Medicine and Physical Culture. 1977; 121-135 [In Bulgarian].

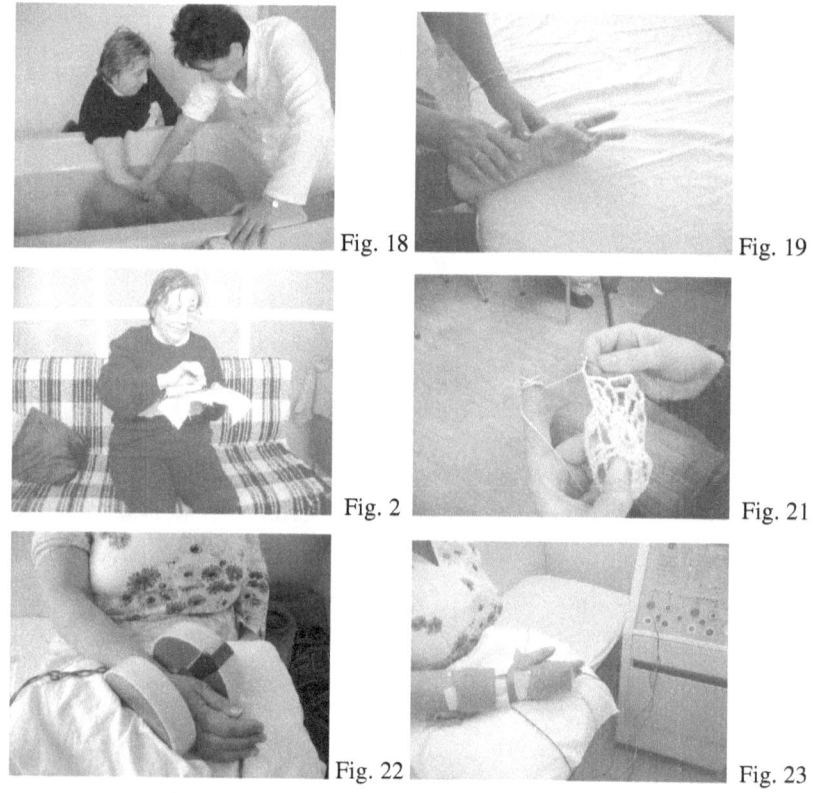

Fig. 18 Fig. 19
Fig. 2 Fig. 21
Fig. 22 Fig. 23

Test for activities of daily living

When starting the physiotherapeutic program all patients were put to the test on activities from everyday life (AEL), prepared in the Centre for Medical Rehabilitation in New York.[1] This test consists of four parts:
- toilet and personal hygiene maintenance,
- activities connected to putting on shoes and clothes,
- activities for preparing food and feeding
- other daily and labour activities.

The assessment is 6-graded (from 0 to 5), and the patients assessed themselves

---
[1] Rusk H. Rehabilitation Medicine. – St. Louis, 1964; 38-49.

following basic activities no matter a dominant limb (DL) or NDL was injured:

- grade 0 when the tested patient cannot perform the activity;
- grade 1 when the tested patient is trying to do the activity but it is necessary to be helped significantly;
- grade 2 when the tested patient is doing the activity, but it is necessary for an assistant to oversee it;
- grade 3 when the tested patient is doing the activity slowly and with limited capacity;
- grade 4 when the tested patient is doing the activity with near normal power, velocity, coordination and durability;
- grade 5 when the tested patient performs the activity normally, with good quality, totally independent;

Signs (+) and (−) are given when marks are not full.[1]

The part for performing **other daily and labour activities** includes: *writing (only for the active hand), opening/closing of a door, opening/closing of a window, locking/unlocking with a key, turning over the pages of a book or a newspaper, lighting a match stick, dealing with a wallet and money, coins counting, using a handkerchief, switching on an electrical lamp, manual washing, hanging out the laundry, ironing, dialing (both a mobile phone and a stationary one).*

We tried to select activities that everybody who suffers from a hand trauma, encounters and finds difficult to handle.

For the performance of those elementary at first sight activities we gave guidelines to patients to ease their self-service, to include the injured limb in without sparing it, but putting a moderate load on it.[2, 3]

- The very first thing a patient should do is to sign a document and when the dominant hand is injured this becomes a complicated task.

---

[1] Karaneshev G, Milcheva D. Methods for diagnostics and examination in remedial gymnastics. − Sofia: National Sport Academy. 1984; 26-73 [In Bulgarian].
[2] Krug G. Occupational Therapy: Evidence-Based Interventions for Stroke. Missouri Medicine. 2009; (106:2):145-149.
[3] Mihaylova N. Occupational Therapy in some degenerative diseases of the motor support apparatus. − In: Topuzov I, editor. Occupational Therapy: II part. − Sofia: RIK Simel. 2008; 68-76 [In Bulgarian].

- Turning over the pages of a book or a newspaper requires good coordination and fine finger movements.
- Dealing with wallet and money requires a precise clutch, especially when counting banknotes.
- When opening a door or a window we recommend that the injured limb is used, no matter whether dominant or non-dominant, in order to train the volume of motion in shoulder and radio-ulnar joint.
- Locking and unlocking using a key requires good side clutch of the dominant limb and enough motion in the radio-ulnar joint.
- Switching on and off a desk lamp or another lighting fixture is an easy activity and is recommendable to be performed with the injured limb no matter whether the latter is dominant or non-dominant.
- Every injured person has now and then to do some hand washing of underwear for instance – then they need to be careful with the temperature of the water not to be too hot or too cold, and to mind not to load too much.
- For hanging out the laundry one needs to have good volume of motion in the shoulder joints in case the wash-lines are stretched at a greater height.
- Ironing is an energy-consuming activity, and patients should be cautious with their overall load. We recommend it to be performed on an ironing board while sitting and with a lighter iron, especially if a dominant limb has been injured, and if it is a non-dominant one, more attention should be paid on not burning the fingers as they are difficult to move.
- Using a stationary phone with buttons is a comparatively easy activity, but if it is with a number dial it often impedes patients, which requires the assistance of the sound limb. Using a mobile phone hinders even more the activity, and then both hands are needed so that the injured holds the phone and the sound one pushes the buttons.

Recovery is reported as the data are processed the results from the first rehabilitation course, the stage right after removal of plaster immobilization and upon finishing the rehabilitation process (usually after second and third rehabilitation course). Usually this period lasts for 2-3 months, and init the time for immobilization is also included (an average of 33 days).

With activities usually performed by the dominant limb that require better coordination of the fingers, more strength in the clutch and enough motion in the radio-ulnar and wrist joints (writing, locking and unlocking with a key, turning over the pages of a newspaper, ironing, using a telephone) immediately after removing the plaster immobilization more difficult patients traumatized dominant limbs, but at the end of the rehabilitation process recover better.

With activities that can be performed equally well by the dominant and the non-dominant limbs (opening/closing of a door or a window, using a handkerchief, switching on an electrical lamp, and hanging out the laundry) not impede patients at the beginning of rehabilitation process.

MEDICAL REHABILITATION AND OCCUPATIONAL THERAPY AFTER MAMESTOMIYA

Over the past years we have seen a significant increase in the number of patients undergoing surgery due to breast cancer (mamectomy). The lowest age of the patients of working age is also decreasing.

The shoulder joint movement capacity of the patients is limited after the surgery as a result of the interruption of the lymph circulation and the formation of keloid scars.[1]

This requires a targeted, full recovery treatment for the patients in order for them to be able to perform their day-to-day activities and be able to return to their active professional and social life within the shortest timeframe possible.[2]

For the goals of our study, at the beginning of the rehabilitation program we measured the shoulder joint movement capacity of the side that underwent surgery based on the standard method of goniometry – SFTR method, where the generally

---

[1] Popov N, Dimitrova E. Kinesitherapy in orthopedic diseases and injuries of the upper limb. – Sofia: NSA – Press. 2007; 295-323 [In Bulgarian].
[2] Ternovoy KS, Kravchenko AA, Leshtinskiy AF. Rehabilitation Therapy in Trauma Locomotory System. – Kiev: Health. 1982; 65-71 [In Russian].

accepted norms for the sagittal plane are S: (flexion – extension) 50° – 0° – 180°, and for the frontal plane F: (abduction – adduction) 180° – 0° – 0°.[1]

Program in Kinesitherapy

The Kinesitherapy method with instructions for day-to-day activities is developed and implemented in Physical and Rehabilitation Medical Clinic since more than 30-th years and begins on the second day after surgery, on the patient's bed in the hospital room. The procedure lasts 7-8 minutes at first and 10-15 minutes at the last few days before the patient is released.[2] The presence of a vacoom-drenage is also allowed (fig. 24).

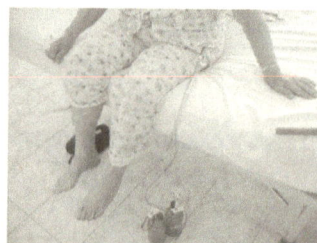

Fig. 24

The *Kinesitherapy program* consists of:

❖ Exercises from a **resting position** (2-3 days after surgery) – isometric contractions of the large muscle groups of the shoulder girdle are performed in the patient's bed in a circulatory system (1:1); active exercises in the shoulder joint with the help of a gymnastics stick; exercises for the shoulder joint, wrist joint and fingers going from the proximal to the distal joints for better lymph drainage. Patients are given instructions for positional therapy, combined with some basic activities regarding dressing up and maintaining personal hygiene (fig. 25-28).[3]

---

[1] Karaneshev G, Milcheva D. Methods for diagnostics and examination in remedial gymnastics. – Sofia: National Sport Academy. 1984; 26-73 [In Bulgarian].
[2] Karaneshev G, Sokolov B, Venova L et al. Edited by G. Karaneshev. Theoty ang methods of remedial gymnastics. – Sofia: Medicine and Physical Culture. 1983; 62-69 [In Bulgarian].
[3] Vasilievoy V. Therapeutic Physical Culture. – Moscow: Medicine. 1970; 119-127 [In Russian].

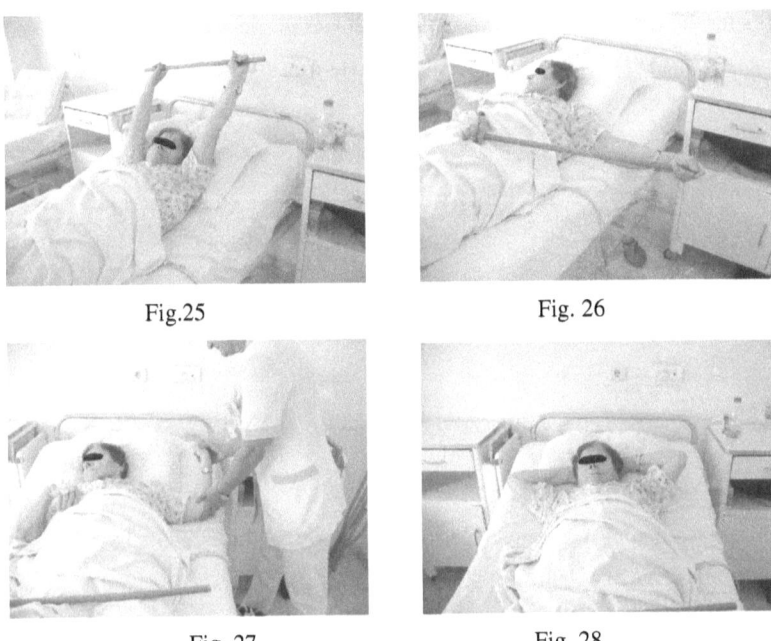

Fig.25

Fig. 26

Fig. 27

Fig. 28

❖ Exercises from a **sitting position** (4-5 days after surgery) – we expand the number and variety of exercises with ones for the neck muscles and the shoulder girdle, along with active exercise for the limbs which are combined with proper breathing and moderate walking[1] (fig. 29, 30);

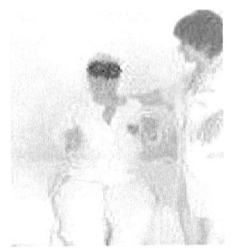

Fig. 29

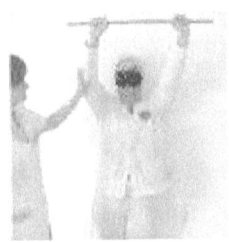

Fig. 30

❖ Exercises from a **standing position** (6-8 days after surgery) – additional

---

[1] Popov N, Dimitrova E. Kinesitherapy in orthopedic diseases and injuries of the upper limb. – Sofia: NSA – Press. 2007; 295-323 [In Bulgarian].

exercises for the limbs and ones with tools (a gymnastic stick) are included, unaided performing of the DtDA - dressing up and moderate walks[1] (fig. 31, 32);

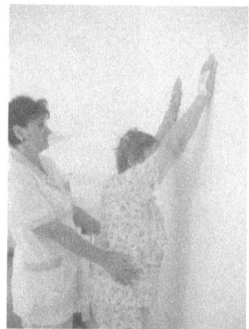
Fig. 31

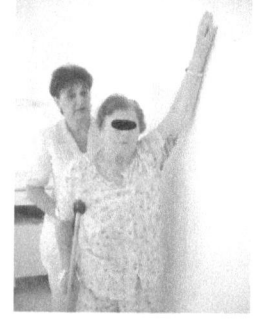
Fig. 32

The rehabilitation program is performed on a daily basis until the patient is released from the surgery ward.

Test Activities of Daily Living
(toilet and personal hygiene)

All patients were put to the test on activities from everyday life (AEL) - prepared in the Centre for Medical Rehabilitation in New York.[2]

The part for **performing toilet and personal hygiene maintenance** includes: *going to the bathroom, hands washing, face washing, tooth brushing, hands/face wiping, hair combing, shaving (for men).*[3]

To help the patients perform these activities more easily, we gave them the following advice:

- To wear clothes which allowed free movements (a night gown) to make going to the bathroom easier;
- When washing their hands, the limb on the non-operated side should

---

[1] Slanchev P, Bonev L, Bankov St. Textbook on Kinesitherapy. – Sofia: Medicine and Physical Culture. 1986; 103-106 [In Bulgarian].
[2] Rusk H. Rehabilitation Medicine. – St. Louis, 1964; 38-49.
[3] Reed K, Sandarson S. Conceps of Occupational therapy. – USA – Lippincott: W & M. 2004; 384-391.

hold the detergent and clean the limb on the side which underwent surgery, after which both limbs are washed under running water;

- When washing the face, the hand on the unaffected side keeps the other one in a supinated position, and splash water to the face as much as possible depending on the patient's ability;
- If the dominant side was the operated one, when brushing teeth this is the hand that is trained, armpit pressed against the body, while brushing itself up and down is helped by full flexibility of the elbow joint, flexion and extension in the wrist joint and head movement;
- Both limbs are used when drying the hands and face, and the hand on the unaffected side dries the other one and helps with the face;
- For combing hair, the limb on the affected side is stimulated regardless whether it's the dominant one or not, as this activity can be easily performed with the non-dominant side as well;
- Shaving is a vital part of men's hygiene and is significantly impaired when the dominant side undergoes surgery, but it still can be done using full flexibility of the elbow joint, flexion and extension in the wrist joint and head rotation;

Undergoing early rehabilitation restores the power and volume of movement of the upper limb which is on the affected side of patients, and it also soothes the pain, prevents the occurrence of lymphoedema and stimulates the ability of self-service.[1]

Patients whose dominant side was operated face bigger difficulties during self-service and maintaining personal hygiene, compared to patients who underwent surgery of the non-dominant side. At the end of the rehabilitation course, shows improvement in patients regardless of the side that underwent surgery.

We observed a genuine improvement in the functional movements of the upper limb which is on the affected side, in the intensity of the pain in the shoulder joint and in the depressive state of the patients caused by the change in their everyday life.

---

[1] Sinaki M. Basic clinical rehabilitation medicine. – Toronto – Philadelphia: W. B. Saunders Co. 1987; 42-51.

Early rehabilitation of patients who underwent mamectomy helps their faster recovery and return to their normal daily activities, in both private and professional aspect. With good cooperation from the patient's side and the performing of the suggested exercise program at home they regain full capacity of their shoulder joint movement on the side which had surgery. Younger patients are released from the surgery ward without any movement limitations and self-service difficulties. The efforts put in early rehabilitations contribute to the improvement of their psychological and emotional state.[1]

MEDICAL REHABILITATION AND OCCUPATIONAL THERAPY IN PATIENTS WITH LESION OF PLEXUS BRACHIALIS

Anatomy, Etiology and Pathogenesis

Plexus brachialis is a net of somatic nerve fibers, extending from the four lower front roots of the spinal column cervical part, and from the first chest nerve (C5-C8 and T1 – fig. 33). The formed plexus goes through the neck, continues to the armpit area through the cervical axillary canal and, branching out to separate periphery nerves, reaches the armpit (brachium), and ends up at the forearm (antebrachium) and the arm (manus). Plexus brachialis is responsible for upper limb muscles motor innervations.

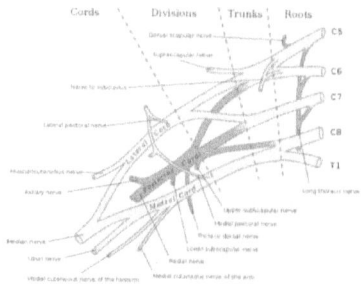

Fig. 33   Topography of the plexus brachialis[2]

---

[1] Pedreti LW, Early MB. Occupational therapy – Practice Skills for Physical Disfunction. Fifth Edition. – USA: St. Louis – Mosby – Elsevier. 2005; 345-367.
[2] http://www.advancedreconstruction.com/brachial-plexus-injuries

Causes for plexus brachialis damage are versatile, and in some cases remain unknown (idiopathica), but mostly result from degenerative and inflammatory processes. Very often the nerve roots are being pressed due to aggravated cervicoarthrosis or hernia discalis cervicalis, but may be inflamed after infectious disease, intocsicathio, immunisathio[1] and other. Pressing mechanically the plexus or a single nerve (cervical rib, tumor process) may also cause nevtitis and paresis.[2]

The close proximity of plexus brachialis to the particularly movable structures of the shoulder girdle is often a precondition for traumatic injuries. Direct trauma and overstretched nerve fibers (birth trauma, luxatio atr. humeroscapularis, fractura claviculae, vulnus scissum, punctum and sclopetatium, mamectomia) are frequent cause for acute damage of plexus brachialis.[3]

A leading symptom in plexithis plexus brachialis's clinical picture is the intensive, burning pain in the shoulder joint area, irradiating to the fingers of the hand and increasing when the head and the upper limbs move.[4] It represents peripheral atrophic torpid paresis or paralysis of the upper limb, depending on the severity and level of damage[5,6] (fig. 34, 35).

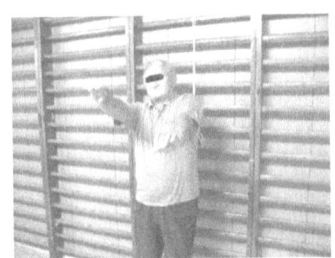
Fig. 34
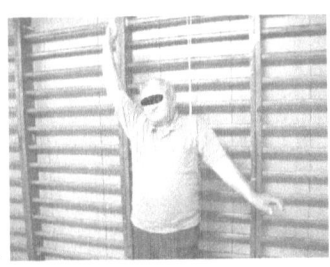
Fig. 35

---

[1] Shy ME. Peripheral neuropathies. In: Goldman L, Schafer AI, eds. Cecil Medicine, 24-th ed. – Philadelphia, Pa: Saunders Elsevier. 2011; 428-431.
[2] Gacheva Y. Ekstsitometrics Electrodiagnostics. – B: Clinical Electrophysiology. Edited by Prof. G. Ganev. – Sofia: Medicine and Physical Culture. 1970; 61-69 [In Bulgarian].
[3] Ensrud E, King JC. Plexopathy-brachial. In: Frontera WR, Silver JK, Rizzo TD, eds. Essentials of Physical Medicine and Rehabilitation, 2-nd ed. – Philadelphia, Pa: Saunders Elsevier. 2008; 134-145.
[4] Ovcharov Vl. Morphology of pain. – B: Pain – pathogenesis and treatment. Edited by P. Shotekov. – Sofia: Leader press. 1998; 146-149 [In Bulgarian].
[5] Bosnev V. Neurovegetative pathology of the hand. – Sofia: Medicine and Physical Culture. 1998; 46-49 [In Bulgarian].
[6] Stucki G, Ewert T, Cieza A. Value and application of the ICF in rehabilitation medicine. Disability and Rehabilitation. 2002; (24):932-938.

Two major types of upper limb dysfunction are distinguished – upper type (Duchen – Erb) and lower type (Dejerin – Klumpke). The pain and the peripheral paresis cause complete or partial immobility of the limb.[1] The patients are not fit for work and meet significant difficulties in performing activities of daily living (ADL).

Diagnosis and Treatment

The disease is diagnosed mainly through anamnesis, with the use of various reflex and manual tests[2], Rö-graphia in order to exclude other pathology and laboratory blood tests for possible inflammations. To establish the injury and damage levels, the developed modern medical diagnostics require use of EMG, in order to exclude a system disease, and MRI and CT for possible spinal pathology.[3]

Treatment of plexithis plexus brachialis is often conservative and is subject to a team of specialists. In severe traumatic conditions, with complete nerve interruption (neurotmesis), urgent operative intervention is a must, for stitching (neuroraphia) or plastica.[4]

Along with symptomatic medication treatment (analgetics, nonsteroidal anti-inflammatory drugs, anticonvulsants, myorelaxants, nivalin, vitamins from the „B" group)[5], it is very important that the injured limb is placed in a suitable orthosis, in order to shorten the plexus and to prevent overstretching of the joint capsule, joints ligaments and tendons in the shoulder joint. Major part of the treatment of this type is appointed to the physical and rehabilitation medicine, and during various periods and stages the means are versatile and individually précised and dosed.[6]

---

[1] Koleva I. Physical analgesia in neurological diseases. Cephalgia. 2006; 8(1):10-21 [In Bulgarian].
[2] Gacheva Y. Ekstsitometrics Electrodiagnostics. – B: Clinical Electrophysiology. Edited by Prof. G. Ganev. – Sofia: Medicine and Physical Culture. 1970; 93-98 [In Bulgarian].
[3] Delank H. Edited by Delank. Neurology. – Sofia: MI Sharov. 1996; 127-131.
[4] Katirji B, Koontz D. Disorders of peripheral nerves. In: Daroff RB, Fenichel GM, Jankovic J, Mazziotta JC, eds. Bradley's Neurology in Clinical Practice, 6-th ed. – Philadelphia, Pa: Saunders Elsevier. 2012; 76-82.
[5] Georgiev I, Bozhinov S. Textbook on Nervous Disease. – Sofia: Medicine and Physical Culture. 1982; 89-104 [In Bulgarian].
[6] Gatev St, Bankov St, Busarov St. Manual for Physical Therapy. – Sofia: Medicine and Physical Culture. 1992; 96-104 [In Bulgarian].

Complex Program in Physiotherapy and Rehabilitation

Depending on the cause, severity of injury and period of recovery, the patients received a series of remedial courses of **complex physio rehabilitation** that include:

- *Electrostimulation* – impulse frequency less than 1 Hz, duration 300-500 ms and pause 3-4 times higher than the impulse, the current is exponential[1, 2];

- *Remedial massage* for maintaining paretic muscle and muscle group trophy; at start, the remedial process is light and gentle, and when the recovery progresses, it gets more energetic and stimulating[3];

- *Kinesitherapy,* aiming to maintain the muscle trophy, to prevent subsequent contractures, to support and stimulate weak and hypotonic muscles and muscle groups[4] (fig. 36-39).

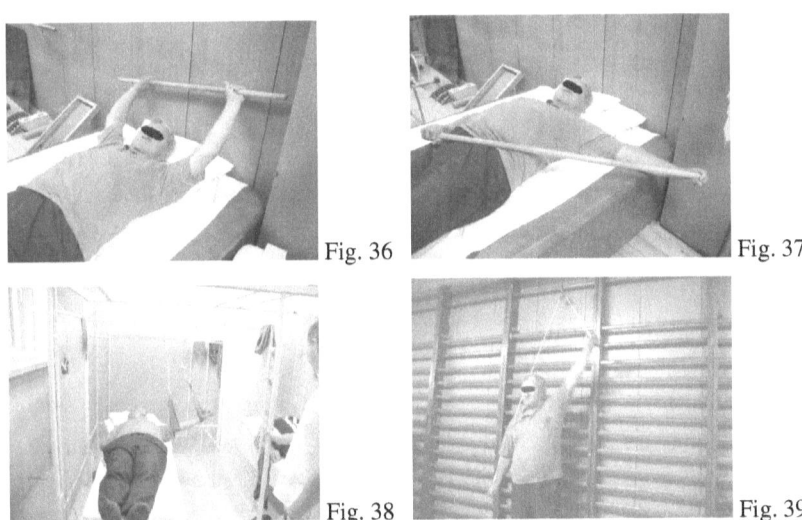

Fig. 36 Fig. 37

Fig. 38 Fig. 39

---

[1] Gatev St, Bankov St, Busarov St. Manual for Physical Therapy. – Sofia: Medicine and Physical Culture. 1992; 165-175 [In Bulgarian].
[2] Schleenbaker RE, Mainous AG. Electromyographic biofeedback for neuromuscular reeducation in the hemiplegic stroke patient: A meta-analysis. Archives of Physical Medicine and Rehabilitation. 1993; 74(2):1301-1304.
[3] Slanchev P, Bonev L, Bankov St. Textbook on Kinesitherapy. – Sofia: Medicine and Physical Culture. 1986; 119-123 [In Bulgarian].
[4] Karaneshev G, Sokolov B, Venova L et al. Edited by G. Karaneshev. Theoty ang methods of remedial gymnastics. – Sofia: Medicine and Physical Culture. 1983; 97-103 [In Bulgarian].

- *Treatment with pre-formed physio factors* – EF with Nivalin (+), 10-15 min, 6-10 mA to assist nerve regeneration; Interference current for pain relief, current frequency 90-100 Hz for 5 min and switching to 1-100 Hz frequency for 10 min; Magnet therapy, that improves the trophy, metabolism, tissue regeneration and has anti inflammatory effect – transverse methodic, 15 min, impulse mode, 200 Oe; Phonophoresis – applied locally, with nonsteroid anti inflammatory means – unstable methodic in the lesion area, 10 min, impulse mode, 800 KHz 0,4-0,6 W/c^{M2}.[1]

- *Ergotherapy* – under the form of guidelines facilitating the ADL, and that include set of practices for maintaining personal hygiene, dressing up and putting shoes on, preparation of food and having meal, various daily and labor activities.[2]

All patients had 4-5 physio rehabilitation remedial courses, duration between 3-4 months and 6 months, and in most severe cases the treatment continued 2 years.[3]

Results from a Clinical Study of Patients with Plexopathy of Plexus Brachialis

The objective of the research is to report the recovery of patients with lesion of plexus brachialis after conducted a complex physio rehabilitation treatment.

Units under observation – 159 patients (86 men and 73 women), age between 29 and 78, with injured plexus brachialis, who have sought physio rehabilitation treatment at the Clinic of Physical Therapy, University Hospital of Pleven, for the period January 2012 – June 2013.

All patients have been diagnosed, with prescribed medication therapy and they have been directed for physio therapy by neurologist. Some of the patients have been admitted for hospital rehabilitation, and other have received ambulatory treatment. From all patients, 53 have damage after a trauma, 71 – root injury due to cervicoarthrosis or hernia discalis cervicalis, 17 have complications after infectious diseases, and the rest 18 patients are of unclear etiology.

---

[1] Gatev St, Bankov St, Busarov St. Manual for Physical Therapy. – Sofia: Medicine and Physical Culture. 1992; 192-198 [In Bulgarian].
[2] Topuzov I. Occupational Therapy. – Sofia: RIK Simel, III part, 2009; 73-79; [In Bulgarian].
[3] Slanchev P, Bonev L, Bankov St. Textbook on Kinesitherapy. – Sofia: Medicine and Physical Culture. 1986; 146-147 [In Bulgarian].

The methods and tests used in the research are: pain assessment – *VAS*; *centimetry*; *MMT* – assessment of upper limb muscle weakness, Vladimir Yanda; *dynamometry* of fist grip; functional test of upper limb – *ADL*.

This test was created by H. Rusk at the Centre of medical rehabilitation – New York[1]. Four stages were included in it: personal grooming and hygiene; putting on shoes and dressing; food preparation and feeding; different social and labor activities. The assessment is 6-graded (from 0 to 5), and the patients assessed themselves following basic activities no matter a dominant or not dominant limb was injured.[2]

During the pain assessment the patients used points from 0 to 20; no pain is indicated by 20 points, and strong, drug-uncontrollable pain is indicated by 0 points. The centimetry of armpit, forearm and through the palm is measured in cm, with linear centimeter tape, and displays presence of edema (marked with "+" sign) or hypertrophy of injured limb (marked with " –" sign), in comparison to the healthy limb. The dynamometry is conducted using a standard dynamometer, completing three trials and registering the best result in kg. This test displays the condition of the forearm muscles and fingers that take part in had grip. All measurements and tests are performed at the beginning of the recovery process, after each rehabilitation course, and at the end of the recovery period; the results are entered in separate file-card for each patient.

The research data have been entered in WIN Excel spreadsheet, and arithmetic mean of all examined patients results from the beginning and from the end of the monitored period have been processed.

The results of the tests we put in a specially developed individual for each patient card and the data processing we did as per Wilcoxon rank test (a statistical method for analysis and distribution of non-parametric data). Processed, the results of the functional test (ADL). Results' significance, for determinations and conclusions has been calculated at $p < 0,05$.

---

[1] Rusk H. Rehabilitation Medicine. – St. Louis, 1964; 38-49.
[2] Karaneshev G, Milcheva D. Methods for diagnostics and examination in remedial gymnastics. – Sofia: National Sport Academy. 1984; 26-73 [In Bulgarian].

In figure 40 are shown the muscles, which are innervated by plexus brachialis.

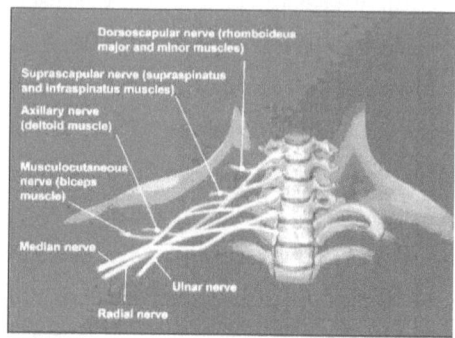

Fig. 40[1]

Figure 41 represents in graphics improvement of tested muscles, innervated by the nerves extended from the plexus brachialis (n. axillaris, n. musculocutaneus, n. radialis, n. medianus, n. ulnaris) at the start of physio rehabilitation treatment and at the end of the recovery period.

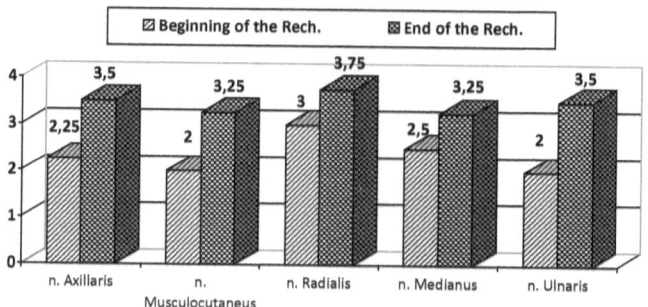

Fig.41 Results MMT muscle innervated by nerves of plexus brachialis at the beginning and end of the recovery process

The VAS pain results, centimetry and dynammetry results are displayed in Table 1; column 1 contains data from the rehabilitation start period, and column 2 – data from the end of the rehabilitation period; column 3 reports the improvement.

---

[1] http://www.aafp.org/afp/2000/1101/p2067.html

Table 1 Results from arithmetic averages of VAS for the pain, centimeters and dynamometers at the beginning and end of the recovery process in patients to the disability of plexus brachialis, grouped depending on the reasons of the lesion

Patient group	Patients with traum. lesion			Patients with disabilities roots			Patients with infectious disabil.			Patients with inflamm. disabil.		
Research	1	2	3	1	2	3	1	2	3	1	2	3
VAS for the Pain	7,9	15,6	7,7	11,7	17,2	5,5	13,4	17,5	4,1	12,3	17,9	5,6
Centim. of the Brachium	-2,3	-0,8	1,5	-1,7	-0,8	0,9	-1,9	-0,7	1,2	-1,2	-0,4	0,8
Centim. of the Anthebrachium	-1,4	-0,5	0,9	-1,1	-0,5	0,6	-1,1	-0,5	0,6	-0,9	-0,4	0,5
Centim. of the Palm	+1,9	+0,5	1,4	+1,1	+0,5	0,6	+0,8	+0,3	0,5	+0,9	+0,3	0,6
Dinamom. Men	9,7	15,6	5,9	11,7	18,4	6,7	12,3	19,6	7,3	10,8	18,7	7,9
Dinamom. Women	2,6	6,8	4,2	5,7	9,8	4,1	6,9	10,2	3,3	6,2	9,6	3,3

Figure 42 shows the test results ADL at the beginning and end of treatment. At the end of the rehabilitation course the Wilcoxon curves were dislocated to the right, which means improvement in the independence of the patients, with both a dominant or not dominant limb was injured and improving their quality of life and work.

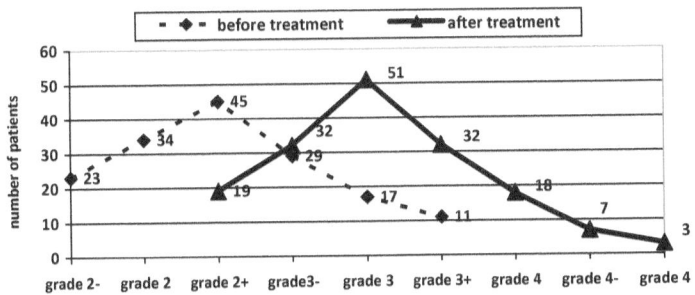

Fig. 42 Curve a Wilcoxon of results of the test ADL from beginning and end of the treatment

The dynamic life of people, multiplied traumatism, unceasing industrial failures, natural calamities and military confrontations lead to increased sick rate of muscle and skeleton system diseases worldwide. We encounter more often problems of individuals in active age, with neuromuscular and disabilities, that should be treated promptly.

A number of publications point out the frequency of plexus brachialis lesion, the affected separate plexus nerves, age limits and the sex ratio.[1] Our research confirmed a numerical superiority of men – 54% of all patients. The reason for injuries in younger age (under 50) is mostly trauma[2], and in older patients (age over 60) is due to degenerative problems, infectious complications or intoxication. In case of mechanically pressed plexus surgery for decompression is required, followed by subsequent rehabilitation program.[3]

The analysis of research derived results confirmed a need for a complex treatment, expressed in a serious medication therapy, combined with systematic, continuous and adequate rehabilitation program. The neurological pain is a leading symptom, and a series of publications suggest therapy with analgetics and anti inflammatory drugs, in order to create optimal precondition for conduct of adequate physio therapy[4]. The medical science is in a constant search for suitable drugs that shall stimulate regeneration of injured peripheral nerves[5], but so far, application of Nivalin, which in severe cases is injected according to a scheme, along with vitamins from the B group and compulsory local application with the help of EE, is indispensable.[6]

The prime importance of applied electrostimulation on injured muscles and muscle groups is indisputable, but often this is not possible due to lack of proper

---

[1] Tsairis P, Dyck PJ, Mulder DW. Natural history of brachial plexus neuropathy. Report on 99 patients. Arch Neurol. 1972; (27):109-117.
[2] http://emedicine.medscape.com/article/1175276-overview
[3] http://www.advancedreconstruction.com/brachial-plexus-injuries
[4] Katirji B, Koontz D. Disorders of peripheral nerves. In: Daroff RB, Fenichel GM, Jankovic J, Mazziotta JC, eds. Bradley's Neurology in Clinical Practice, 6-th ed. – Philadelphia, Pa: Saunders Elsevier. 2012; 114-119.
[5] Yiancheva S, Milanov I, Georgiev D, Shotekov P. Motor activity. In: Yiancheva S, editor. Neurology – General neurology. – Stara Zagora: College. 1998; 105-109 [In Bulgarian].
[6] Georgiev I, Bozhinov S. Textbook on Nervous Disease. – Sofia: Medicine and Physical Culture. 1982; 141-147 [In Bulgarian].

equipment and trained staff in most of the existing physiotherapy medical establishments in our country.[1] In such cases a reliable option is the professionally conducted systematic kinesiotherapy that influences the reduced muscle power of the whole upper limb. Analytic, passive, aided and active exercises for the upper limb joints are applied; also manual techniques and mobilization of periphery joints, special techniques from the proprioceptive neuromuscular facilitation of Kabat, suspension exercises for the muscles that move the shoulder joint within the front and sagittal plane, exercises with and on apparatuses for upper limbs, preventing contractures, pull therapy for strengthening weak and hypotrophy muscles.[2,3]

Recognizing the functional recovery of the upper limb, improved self-service of patients, performance of various labor activities and return to independent, full-value life is the objective of the specialists that conduct the **rehabilitation at first hand**.[4]

Improvement of measured indexes is registered in all patients under observation, and the duration of the treatment is dependent on cause, severity and level of injury of plexus brachialis.

In order to achieve good results in rehabilitation of patients with injured plexus brachialis and improved abilities for ADL, crucial significance have timely diagnosis, good medication therapy and early start of complex physio rehabilitation program that includes electrotherapy, electrostimulation, kinesiotherapy and ergotherapy. The good results come slowly and with difficulties, but the patients' quality of life and labor is being improved significantly.

---

[1] Berner YN, Kimchi OL, Spokoiny V, Finkeltov B. The effect of electrical stimulation treatment on the functional rehabilitation of acute geriatric patients with stroke – a preliminary study. Archives of Gerontology and Geriatrics. 2004; (39):125-132.
[2] Slanchev P, Bonev L, Bankov St. Textbook on Kinesitherapy. – Sofia: Medicine and Physical Culture. 1986; 152-154 [In Bulgarian].
[3] Shiflett S, Nayak S, Bid C et al. The effect of reiki treatments on functional recovery in patients in poststroke rehabilitation: a pilot study. The Journal of Alternative and Complementary Medicine. Mary Ann Liebert. 2002; 8(6):755-763.
[4] Trombly CA. Occupational Therapy for Physical Dysfunction. – Boston – Baltimore – Philadelphia – Hong-Kong – London – New York – Sydney – Tokyo: Williams & Wilkins. 1996; 121-127.

OCCUPATIONAL THERAPY IN PATIENTS WHO SUFFER FROM CEREBRAL VASCULAR DISEASE

Bulgaria is in a leading position in the world as regards morbidity, sick rate and mortality of brain vascular disease (BVD).[1] Younger patients are being affected in recent years. Main consequences were heavy disability – motor disorders, difficulties with self service, professional and social dys-adaptation, deteriorating quality of life, depressions.[2, 3] About 80% of the survivors from a brain vascular incident overcome the dependence of other people's help, about 26% from them were diagnosed with vascular dementia and impairment of communication, about 20% were confined to their bed.[4, 5, 6]

Causes for this epidemic of BVD are increasing the frequency of risk factors such as atherosclerosis of the brain vessels, arterial hypertension, chronic ischemic heart disease, overweight, diabetes mellitus, malnutrition, alcohol abuse and smoking, chronic stress, etc.

The physical and rehabilitation medicine is of vital importance for optimal recuperation and saving self-dependence ability achieved in patients with consequences of BVD, as in the beginning of the rehabilitation process the stress is mainly on everyday activities.[7, 8, 9]

---

[1] Georgiev I, Bozhinov S. Textbook on Nervous Disease. – Sofia: Medicine and Physical Culture. 1982; 164-166 [In Bulgarian].

[2] Gencheva N. Classificational system for manual capacity (MAGS) in children with cerebral palsy. Sport i Nauka. 2011; (1):60-65 [In Bulgarian].

[3] Yiancheva S, Milanov I, Georgiev D, Shotekov P. Motor activity. In: Yiancheva S, editor. Neurology – General neurology. – Stara Zagora: College. 1998; 204-227 [In Bulgarian].

[4] Koleva I. The bulgarian neurorehabilitation school and the international classification of functioning, disability and health (icf): integrating icf requirements into clinical practice. J. Biomed. Clin. Res. 2009; 2(1):8-18 [In Bulgarian].

[5] Logan PA, Gladman JRF, Avery A, Walker MF, Dyas J, Groom L. Randomised Controlled Trial of an Occupational Therapy Intervention to Increase Outdoor Mobility after Stroke. BMJ. 2004; (25):1136-1139.

[6] World Health Organization. International Classification of Functioning. Disability and Health (ICF), WHO, Geneva, 2001.

[7] Hannecke van Bruggen. Occupational therapy (ergotherapy) – philosophy, objectives and methodology. Rehabilitation Medicine and the Quality of Life. 2007; (2):16 [In Bulgarian].

[8] Kostadinov D, Gacheva Y, Tsvetanova L. Manual Physical Therapy. – Sofia: Medicine and Physical Culture. Tom 1, 1989; 103-106 [In Bulgarian].

[9] Mollova K, Paskaleva R. Rehabilitation activities in patients with motor dosturbancer. Collection materials of International cientific conferention – Stara Zagora's bads. 2009; 32-35 [In Bulgarian].

Results from a Clinical Study in Patients suffering from Cerebral Vascular Disease

The aim of the our research is to investigate, follow up and report on the recovery level of the most important activities in everyday life (AEL), namely the ability for food preparation and feeding in patients with BVD.

During the period 2010-2011 year 61 patients diagnosed with consequences of BVD (23 women and 38 men, between 37 – 75 years old), have passed through the department of hospital rehabilitation and the clinic of physical medicine and rehabilitation.

A right-side paresis had found in 37 of the patients, and 34 of them were with NDL affected (fig. 43). The side of the paretic limb was of decisive importance for AEL.

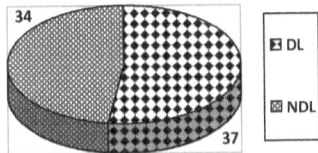

Fig. 43 Distribution of the patients with injured DL and NDL

All of the patients were following a **physical rehabilitation program** consistent with their individual status. It generally includes: *kinesitherapy; labor therapy (occupational therapy and AEL), electrotherapy.*[1,2]

All patients at the beginning of the rehabilitation course were tested for AEL. This test was created by H. Rusk at the Centre of medical rehabilitation – New York: toilet and personal hygiene maintenance; activities for preparing food and feeding.[3]

---

[1] Karaneshev G, Sokolov B, Venova L et al. Edited by G. Karaneshev. Theoty ang methods of remedial gymnastics. – Sofia: Medicine and Physical Culture. 1983; 149-152 [In Bulgarian].
[2] Slanchev P, Bonev L, Bankov St. Textbook on Kinesitherapy. – Sofia: Medicine and Physical Culture. 1986; 246-247 [In Bulgarian].
[3] Rusk H. Rehabilitation Medicine. – St. Louis, 1964; 38-49.

These are activities from everyday life that every person is confronted with. The results of the tests were recorded in a specially developed individual patient card.

Test Activities of Daily Living
(activities for preparing food and feeding)

The part for **activities for preparing food and feeding** includes: *set in/pull out a plug, turning on/off a heater switch, turn on/off a water tab, washing up kitchen utensils, pouring and drinking liquids in a cup, serving the food in a plate, feeding with a spoon, feeding with a fork, cutting products with a knife, cleaning the table.*

- Using the switches of a heater requires significant strength for clutching and enough volume motion in the radio-ulnar joint. In the beginning of the rehabilitation process this is difficult, even impossible, for many patients. This situation requires considerable support of the healthy limb, especially when the DL is paretic, grasping the clutch and supporting the locomotion for turning over the switch.

- Switching on and especially switching off require considerable strength of the palmar grasp, acting of the healthy limb is needed, while the paretic limb supports the contact (fig.44).

- The turning on/off of tab water is not so difficult an activity, especially if they are with a pick up/down nozzle, but if traditional, with hand clutches that turn, they also require considerable strength and enough motion in the radio-ulnar joint. We recommend the patients to include the paretic limb (if possible) and to support the motion with the healthy limb (fig. 45).

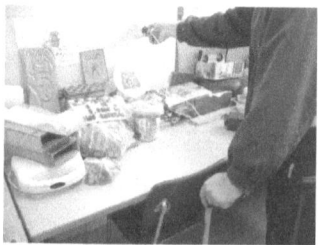
Fig. 44

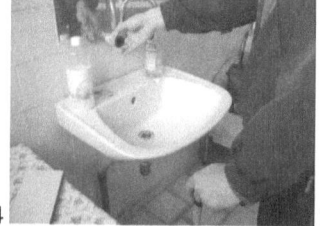
Fig. 45

- When washing plates one must be very careful, if plates are fragile. Beware of slipping, breaking down and eventually cutting themselves. The plate must be held with the healthy limb while the paretic one is doing the washing with gel and sponge; and for rinsing the activities of the hands may be changed.
- When pouring liquids in the glass, the patients must keep in mind the weight of the bottle. It should not be too heavy. The intact hand mainly takes the weight, while the paretic one is only supporting pouring into cup. We recommend turning on and off of the stopper to be performed with the paretic limb (if possible), and if needed the healthy one supports the activity (fig. 46).
- When drinking liquids from a glass we recommend the use of the paretic limb, but taking in consideration the weight and material which the cup is made of – not too heavy, of anti-fragile materials and with the biggest possible diameter. This stimulates the cylindrical clutch and trains extensor muscles of the fingers and the wrist (fig. 47).

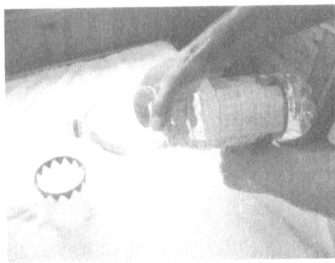
Fig. 46

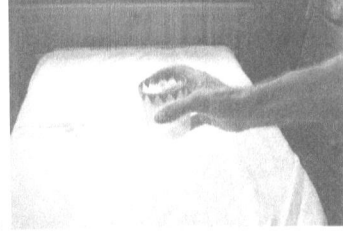
Fig. 47

- When the DL was affected the pouring of food in a plate and feeding becomes significantly difficult. In this case we recommend using a deeper food plate, placed on the plot of the table and then the paretic limb slowly and carefully moves to it. If not impossible to perform this activity by the DL, in the beginning of the recovering process it has be perform with the intact one.
- In the beginning of the recuperation the patients with injured DL are advised to feed themselves with the healthy limb, in order not to be additionally

depressed, then gradually to include the paretic one. We recommend the injured limb to hold a piece of bread, a spoon with non-liquid food or a fork, the clutch in most cases being in position pronation of the ante brachium.

- When patients are using a knife, they should be very careful. A person might have difficulties with NDL and he/she may injure by accident the paretic limb. So the knife should be at a distance from the food fixed by the paretic limb. The food must not to be too hard (frozen meet, butter) and must be positioned on a non-slipping surface. If the NDL is injured, the attention of the patient should be towards its fixing role – if there is enough strength to hold the cutting object and to keep in mind his/her status (fig. 48).

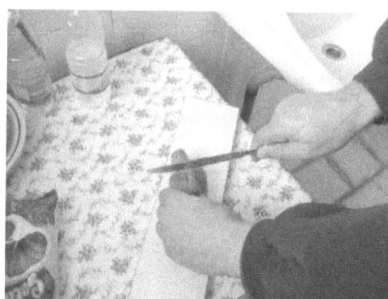

Fig. 48

- In the process of cleaning the table with both limbs – one of them takes the cleaning object and the other – the kitchen spade. The activity of both hands can be changed. The affected limb has a supportive function.

Test results ADL represented by Wilcoxon rank test – a statistical method for analyzing of the non-parametrical data and distribution.

On figure 49 we have exposed curve of the Wilcoxon from the results in the activity *„Preparing food and feeding"* in all patients in the beginning and at the end of the first rehabilitation course. Receiving a double-peaked Wilcoxon's curve in some of the research activities was that patients with paretic DL had bigger difficulties in preparing food and feeding, than those with paretic NDL.

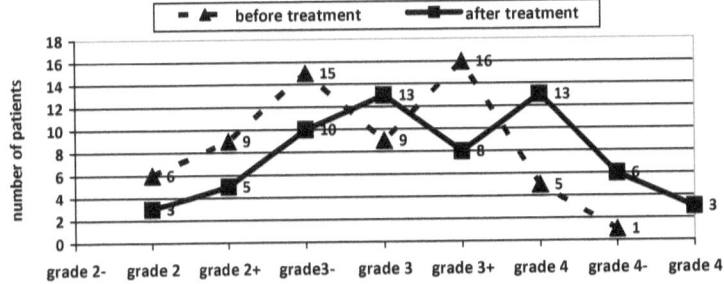

Fig. 49 Results in the first group ADL „Preparing food and feeding" in the beginning and in the end of the rehabilitation course

Test Activities of Daily Living
(toilet and personal hygiene)

The part for **performing toilet and personal hygiene maintenance** includes: *using the toilet, washing one's hands and face, brushing of teeth, wiping of hands/face, combing the hair, shaving with a razor, cutting nails, showering.*[1,2]

Doing these at first sight elementary activities are found difficult by patients [3], so we need to facilitate them and recommend:

- Wearing larger clothes (skirt or sportswear with an elastic band) to be easier visiting the toilet;
- When the patient is washing his/her hands, the healthy limb is holding the washing gel and putting it on the paretic, after that the hands are rinsed under running water;
- For washing the face - the healthy hand supports the injured one in a position of suppination (as far as possible), in order water to be splashed on the face;
- If the dominant limb is injured, it is the one that has to be trained for teeth brushing, and the ante brachium must be in a neutral position and the up-down

---
[1] Topuzov I. Occupational Therapy. – Sofia: RIK Simel, III part, 2009; 213-224 [In Bulgarian].
[2] Hansen RA, Atchison B. Conditions in Occupational Therapy. – Baltimore: Williams & Wilkins. 1993; 38-43.
[3] Petkova I. Interactive methods in educators' qualification, Qualy educayion for all through improving teacher training. Paradigma. 2010; 214-216 [In Bulgarian].

movement when brushing the teeth is supported by the shoulder joint – flexion and extension in adduction;

- If the paretic limb is non dominant, the palmar clutch must be trained for putting tooth-paste on the brush;
- For drying up hands and face both hands are used, the healthy one drying the injured and supporting it for the face;
- Hair styling can be done with the healthy limb, no matter if it is DL or not, this activity can be performed comparatively easy by NDLs;
- At men shaving is a basic part of the personal hygiene and is very difficult with a paretic DL, but it is not impossible if there is a palmar clutch and the activity is supported by the shoulder joint. That includes rotation of the head to compensate for the absence of fine movements of the fingers and flexion and extension in the wrist joint;
- For cutting the nails a precise clutch is necessary, as well as enough strength of the clutch, good motion in wrist and radio ulnar joints, and significant coordination of the movements. The above makes this activity very difficult to perform, especially if the NDL is injured at the beginning of the rehabilitation process (it is useful for patient to use a nail-cutter and orientate the nail towards the appropriate clutch of the paretic limb);
- Taking a bath (shower) is a complex activity, which requires more attention and efforts on the patient's side. The most important thing is prevention of slipping and falling down in the bathroom, thus the patient must be seated during the procedure.

For performing activities of daily living is essential that the side of paresis – of the dominant upper limb or not dominant upper limb. This required the separation of patients into two groups – patients with paresis of the dominant limb and patients with paresis of the not- dominant limb.

The survey included patients are in Stage IV Bryunstryom (scale for determining the functional status of patients with hemiparesis).

Figure 50 presents the curve of Wilcoxon, obtained from the averages of the all the activities included in the Test Activities of Daily Living (toilet and personal hygiene). The curve formed two peaks, which means that there are activities that prevent more patients, and others – less.

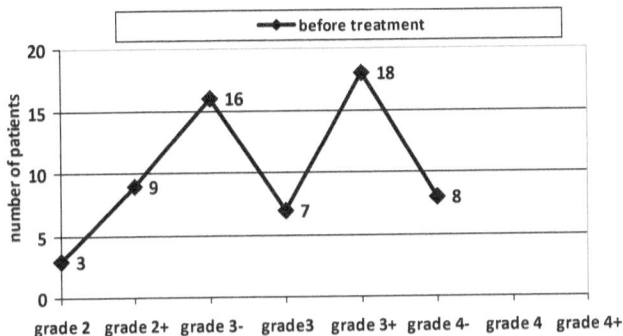

Fig. 50 Results from the ADL „Toilette and supporting of personal hygiene" in the beginning of the rehabilitation course

It had tested activities be divided into two groups – **first**, involving concrete activities that make it difficult at greater patient (*using the toilet, shaving with a razor, cutting nails, showering*) and **second** a more accessible for execution activities (*washing one's hands and face, brushing of teeth, wiping of hands/face, combing the hair*).

Table 2 shows the test data ADL by activity, at the beginning and end of the rehabilitation course and patients with paretic DL and NDL.

Table 2 Results shows the test data ADL by activity

Type of Activity *First group activities*	Patients with paretic DL		Patients with paretic NDL	
	Beginning of the reh. course	*End of the reh. course*	*Beginning of the reh. course*	*End of the reh. course*
Using the WC	2-	3	3-	4-
Shaving with a razor (for men)	2	3-	3	4-
Cutting nails	2-	2+	3-	3+
Showering	2	3-	2+	3+
Second group activit.				
washing of hands	3-	3+	3+	4
washing of face	2+	3	3	4-
brushing of teeth	2+	3+	4	4+
wiping of hands/face	3	4-	4+	5-
combing the hair	3-	3+	4	5-

Figure 51 shows the improvement results in the **first** group activities of groups patients at the beginning and end of the rehabilitation course.

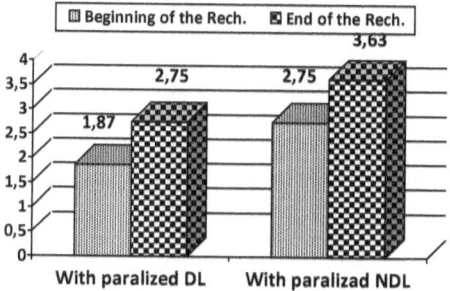

Fig. 51 Results in the first group activities of groups patients at the beginning and end of the rehabilitation course

Figure 52 shows the improvement results in the **second** group activities of groups patients at the beginning and end of the rehabilitation course.

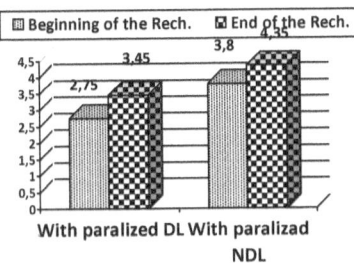

Fig. 52 Results in the second group activities of groups patients at the beginning and end of the rehabilitation course

In the available publications researches are related to functional recovery of brain functions after a stroke, its mechanism still not completely known.[1,2]

It is known that in the basis of a complex physiotherapy and rehabilitation program for patients with post-stroke hemiparesis (neurorehabilitation) is the kinesiotherapy procedure.[3,4] The treatment through movement is expressed in performing a series of active physical exercises, special methods of Bobat[5] and Kabat[6], stage-by-stage verticalization, exercises for balance and coordination, training to move using auxiliary device (locomotion).[7]

To subdue the spasm of the paretic muscle groups, a number of relax techniques and devices from the healing massage are suitable[8], in combination with proper medication therapy (myorelaxants) and passive exercises to prevent contractures, mainly at the shoulder, wrist and ankle joints of paretic extremities. The

---

[1] Delank H. Edited by Delank. Neurology. – Sofia: MI Sharov. 1996; 202-208.
[2] Titynova E. Brain reorganization after a stroke. Neurorehabilitation. 2008; 2(2):22-26 [In Bulgarian].
[3] Karaneshev G, Sokolov B, Venova L et al. Edited by G. Karaneshev. Theoty ang methods of remedial gymnastics. – Sofia: Medicine and Physical Culture. 1983; 188-201 [In Bulgarian].
[4] Paskaleva R. Kinesitherapy motivating role in the fight against obesity. Prevention and Rehabilitation. 2011; (1):23-29 [In Bulgarian].
[5] Paci M. Physiotherapy based on the Bobath concept for adults with post-stroke hemiplegia; A review of effectiveness studies. Journal of Rehabilitation Medicine. 2003; (35):2-7.
[6] Hiraoka K. Rehabilitation effort to improve upper extremity function in post-stroke patients: A meta-analysis. Journal of Physical Therapy Science. 2001; (13):5-9.
[7] Krakauer JW. Motor learning: Its relevance to stroke recovery and neurorehabilitation. Current Opinion in Neurology. 2006; (19):84-90.
[8] Mok E and Woo CP. Slow stroke massage helps stroke patients. Complementary Therapy Nurse Midwifery. 2004; (4):209-216.

healing massage is introduction to the kinesiotherapy procedure, to relax spastic muscles or to stimulate weak and torpid muscle groups.

Researches reveal that about 80% of patients, who suffered cerebrovascular incident, manage to recover their independent walk. As for the upper extremities, about 30% cope with everyday tasks and only 15% recover functionally their upper extremity.[1] In most of the patients with hemiparesis we can see hemiparetic shoulder, that, as a result from weak shoulder muscle system, overstretched muscle tendons, joint capsule or myogenic contraction, a strong pain appears when the shoulder joint is moved. In such cases shall be conducted a number of electrical healing procedures that influence the muscle trophy (impulse magnet field), reduce pain (interference therapy), and, assisted with phonophoresis, shall be applied nonsteroid anti-inflammatory pain-relief drug.[2]

To achieve a maximum possible independency of patients, the home environment often needs remodeling and adaptation to facilitate the daily routine and to prevent incidents (falling down, strikes). The flooring, especially in the bathroom, is very important (slipping, stumbling).[3, 4]

Except for the physical recovery of patients with cerebrovascular disease, their psychic and mental state is of importance too. Any hobby that may divert patient's attention from their health issues has stimulating effect on their general physical and psychic state.[5, 6] Treatment through labor tasks (labor therapy)[7] is known since ancient times. Nowadays it is successfully applied as well, to help recovering lost functions of upper extremities or to favorably influence psychic and emotional state,

---

[1] Legg LA, Drummond AE, Langhorne P. Occupational therapy for patients with problems in activities of daily living after stroke. Cochrane Database of Systematic Reviews. 2006; (4):583-585.
[2] Busarov St. Basis of the medicine-social rehabilitation. – Sofia: Medicine and Physical Culture. 1982, 92-95 [In Bulgarian].
[3] Trombly CA. Occupational Therapy for Physical Dysfunction. – Boston – Baltimor – Philadelphia – Hong-Kong – London – New York – Sydney – Tokyo: Williams & Wilkins. 1996; 216-232.
[4] Vacheva D, Simeonova V, Stamenov B. The Recovery Detection of Daily and Labor Activities in the Everyday Life in Patients who Suffered from Cerebral Vascular Disease. Acta Med. Bulg. 2013; XL(2):46-52.
[5] Hansen RA, Atchison B. Conditions in Occupational Therapy. – Baltimore: Williams & Wilkins. 1993; 112-134.
[6] Steultjens EMJ, Dekker J, Bouter LM, Van de Ness JCM, Cup EHC, Van den Ende CHM. Occupational Therapy for stroke patients: A systematic review. Stroke. 2003; (34):676-687.
[7] Legg LA, Drummond AE, Langhorne P. Occupational therapy for patients with problems in activities of daily living after stroke. Cochrane Database of Systematic Reviews. 2006; (4):583-585.

under the form of interesting labor therapy (hobby). The complex physiorehabilitation program we conduct includes labor therapy – the patients work with yarn, sewing cotton, textile and plastic material according to their preferences and in compliance with individual abilities of each patient. Latham et al. (2006)[1] confirm that for patients who practice labor therapy and ergotherapy in the long run there is less possibility to aggravate in daily routine and is more possible to be independent in their ability to cope with toilet and maintain personal hygiene.

Treatment of patients with post-stroke hemiparesis is done step by step, for a long period. After getting over the acute period of treatment at intensive care neurology clinic and conducted early rehabilitation program, in order to verticalize the patients and train them to walk using auxiliary device and to self-service, a long period of systematically conducted rehabilitation follows.[2] It is a practice with such patients to go through some courses in hospital environment, then through continuous ambulatory physiorehabilitation treatments, and the means of the physical and the rehabilitation medicine are in line with the specifics of each case. The aim of all rehabilitation courses is the maximum functional recovery of paretic extremities and most of all, achievement of independent everyday life of the patient.

We observed significant positive influence on the functional mobility of the paretic limbs, the intensity of the pain of the humero-scapular joint and lowering of the depressive disorders in patients as a result of the improvement of the quality of life – being more independent.

For achieving better results in the rehabilitation of patients with consequences of BVD and enhancing the ability for self-service of significant importance was the early initiation of the rehabilitation and including labor activities and elements of ELA, given as instructions. The functional occupational therapy stimulates the patients' independence and facilitates their recovery to normal everyday life and

---

[1] Latham NK, Jette DU, Coster W et al. Occupational therapy activities and intervention techniques for clients with stroke in six rehabilitation hospitals. American Journal of Occupational Therapy. 2006; 60(4):369-378.
[2] Walker MF, Gladman JRF, Lincoln NB, Siemonsma P, Whiteley T. A randomised con-trolled trial of occupational therapy for stroke patients not admitted to hospital. Lancet 1999; (354):278-280.

social activity.

MEDICAL REHABILITATION AND OCCUPATIONAL THERAPY AMONG PATIENTS WITH ARTHROPLASTIC HIP JOINT

Replacement of a painful or anatomically and functionally disabled joint with a superficial one turns out to be an unquestionable progress by the bone-joint surgery worldwide.[1] Orthopedic biomechanics and biochemistry that work on issues of durability and acceptability of endoprosthesis material by the organism, contributed for this success too.

The motor regimen of the patient is a crucial criterion for successful prosthesis of pelvic and femoral joints; it not only has motor function but also supporting and bearing function.[2] A number of risk factors exist, for mechanical loosening or luxation of the joint prosthesis, and the patient shall be informed and trained to lead a proper life.[3]

Program in Kinesitherapy and Training Walking Assistive Devices

The complex therapy method with instruction for everyday life tasks[4, 5] starts on the second day after surgery, on the patient's bed, in the room (after drainage is removed). The extremity that underwent surgery is treated via special splint, in a slight abduction (fig. 53). Isometric exercises are included, for the large muscle groups around the pelvic, in order to pump out the post-operation swelling of the whole extremity, active exercises for the healthy extremity, mobilization of the knee-cap (the patella dance) of the extremity that underwent surgery (fig. 54), and

---

[1] Takov E, Tivchev P, Ivanov V. The fractures – diagnostic and treatment. – Sofia: Venel. II part, 1996; 305-328 [In Bulgarian].
[2] Kalchev I, Morova E. Kinesiology. – Sofia: University "Sv. Kliment Ohridski". 1993; 107-129 [In Bulgarian].
[3] Ternovoy KS, Kravchenko AA, Leshtinskiy AF. Rehabilitation Therapy in Trauma Locomotory System. – Kiev: Health. 1982; 103-111 [In Russian].
[4] Karaneshev G, Sokolov B, Venova L et al. Edited by G. Karaneshev. Theoty ang methods of remedial gymnastics. – Sofia: Medicine and Physical Culture. 1983; 217-223 [In Bulgarian].
[5] Slanchev P, Bonev L, Bankov St. Textbook on Kinesitherapy. – Sofia: Medicine and Physical Culture. 1986; 268-269 [In Bulgarian].

assisted exercises for bending of knee and pelvic-femoral joints, in turns with active exercises for ankle joints and toes.

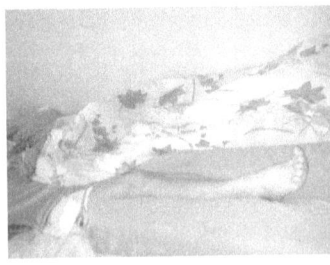
Fig. 53

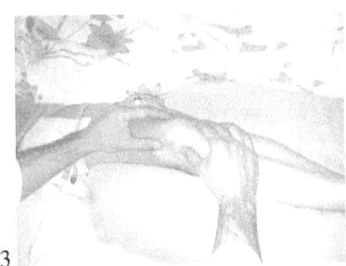
Fig. 54

On day 2-3 after surgery the patient is verticalized (fig. 55) and is trained to walk using auxiliary devices (two crutches), and **they shall be adjusted individually** – as the patient stands (the weight is taken completely by the healthy extremity; the extremity that underwent surgery shall only touch the floor with entire foot), crutches are under the armpit (shoulders not raised), and slightly pointed ahead, at the width of the shoulders; the grips shall be at the level of trochanters (elbow joint is bended at 30°) (fig. 56).

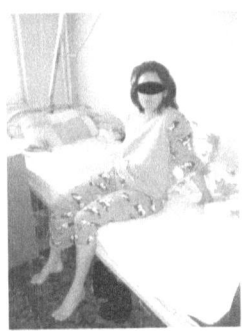
Fig. 55

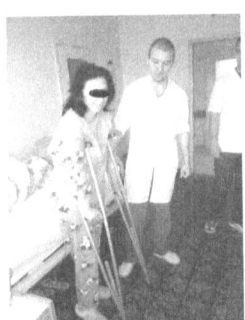
Fig. 56

When **training to walk** with crutches is conducted, there shall be preliminary information on how much shall the operated extremity be loaded (according to the instructions of the attending doctor orthopedist and traumatologist). In the beginning of the rehabilitation process the endoprosthesis extremity shall be spared at maximum, but it doesn't mean that the patient shall jump on one leg. The training to walk properly requests this sequence[1,2]: starting position – the patient lies on his back in the bed; he raises his body and sits in the bed with stretched legs, then carefully sits in the bed and lets the legs down, feet reaching the floor; then the patient takes the crutches, and, pressing the grips, lifts the pelvic and stands up; the body weight is completely on the healthy extremity, and the operated extremity is in a slight abduction; the crutches are placed under the armpit and the patient stands for a few seconds, in order to feel the support of the crutches (the orthostatic reaction is trained).

Walking is done by placing the crutches simultaneously ahead, the body weight taken by the healthy leg, then the operated leg steps at the crutches' level, without going farther ahead; the body weight is transferred on the crutches and a next step is done with the healthy leg, without loading the operated one, and then the movements are repeated again. The sequence of walking with two auxiliary devices is „crutches" – „ill leg" – „healthy leg".

The procedure starts from 7-8 minutes duration, and shall reach 10-15 minutes at discharge day (usually 2 days after operation stitches are removed).

The kinesitherapeutic program, conducted at the early post-surgery period, for patients with endoprosthesis of pelvic-femoral joints contributed to early verticalization of the patient, influences the pain, restores independency and stimulates self-servicing.

A reliable, favorable influence of the functional mobility of the operated leg, pain intensity and decrease of patients' depressive state due to more independent life are monitored.

Early rehabilitation of patients with plastic repair of pelvic-femoral joints allows for faster return to an independent mobility regimen, in home environment.

---

[1] Mihaylova N. Occupational Therapy in some degenerative diseases of the motor support apparatus. – In: Topuzov I, editor. Occupational Therapy: II part. – Sofia: RIK Simel. 2008; 153-155 [In Bulgarian].
[2] Paskaleva R. Kinesitherapy motivating role in the fight against obesity. Prevention and Rehabilitation. 2011; (1):23-29 [In Bulgarian].

With a good cooperation on behalf of the patient and execution of suggested mobility recovery program in home environment, functional recovery and return to previous way of living are achieved, especially when endoprosthesis is placed after fracture.

Efforts made for conducting the early rehabilitation leads to stabilization of the psycho-emotional state of patients. This is necessary to overcome a lengthy period of recovery and use of aids.

Conclusion

It is not yet universally accepted definition of disability and quality of life. Disability is any loss or abnormality of psychological, physiological function or anatomical structure. Disability is any restriction or complete loss of the ability to perform some activity in a normal manner. The focus is on the ability to perform activities.

Around the world there are millions of people with disabilities. According to statistics, 10-20% of the population in each country has a limited performance in result of some type of disability. This percentage continues to increase because of low health culture, malnutrition in childhood, insufficient healthcare provided, the aging of the population, civilian and military conflicts.

Persons with disabilities have special needs. As for the professional engagement – people with disabilities are unemployed 3 times more often than other. The attitude of state institutions for persons with disabilities and people with different capabilities changes constantly. Modern concepts with are in the direction social integration – life with others on equal rights and equal opportunities. Integration is a viable only upon completeness on both sides, only conscious and open position of acceptance, depending on of the socio-cultural norms.

We consider that the result of the complex fisiorehabilitation and occupational therapy program, we have improved the quality of life for our patients who have various motor deficiencies.

References
1. Alexander A.H. Bilateral traumatic dislokation of the distal radioulnar joint, ulna dorsal. – B: Case report and review of the literature. Clin Orthop. 1977; 129-238.
2. AOTA Council on Standards. Occupational therapy – its definition and function. Amer. J. Occup. Therapy. 1972; (26): 204-205.
3. Berner YN, Kimchi OL, Spokoiny V, Finkeltov B. The effect of electrical stimulation treatment on the functional rehabilitation of acute geriatric patients with stroke – a preliminary study. Archives of Gerontology and Geriatrics. 2004; (39):125-132.
4. Bosnev V, Matev I. Disease of the hand. – Sofia: Medicine and Physical Culture. 1989; 174-175; 230-240 [In Bulgarian].
5. Bosnev V. Neurovegetative pathology of the hand. – Sofia: Medicine and Physical Culture. 1998; 46-49 [In Bulgarian].
6. Busarov St. Basis of the medicine-social rehabilitation. – Sofia: Medicine and Physical Culture. 1982, 92-95 [In Bulgarian].
7. Delank H. Edited by Delank. Neurology. – Sofia: MI Sharov. 1996; 127-131; 202-208.
8. Ensrud E, King JC. Plexopathy-brachial. In: Frontera WR, Silver JK, Rizzo TD, eds. Essentials of Physical Medicine and Rehabilitation, 2-nd ed. – Philadelphia, Pa: Saunders Elsevier. 2008; 134-145.
9. Gacheva Y. Ekstsitometrics Electrodiagnostics. – B: Clinical Electrophysiology. Edited by Prof. G. Ganev. – Sofia: Medicine and Physical Culture. 1970; 61-69; 93-98 [In Bulgarian].
10. Gatev St, Bankov St, Busarov St. Manual for Physical Therapy. – Sofia: Medicine and Physical Culture. 1992; 96-104; 165-175; 192-198 [In Bulgarian].
11. Gencheva N. Classificational system for manual capacity (MAGS) in children with cerebral palsy. Sport i Nauka. 2011; (1):60-65 [In Bulgarian].
12. Georgiev I, Bozhinov S. Textbook on Nervous Disease. – Sofia: Medicine and Physical Culture. 1982; 89-104; 141-147; 164-166 [In Bulgarian].
13. Hamonet CL, Heuleu JN. Rééducation fonctionnelle et réadaptation. – Paris – New York – Barcelona – Milan: Masson. 1998; 164-168.
14. Hannecke van Bruggen. Occupational therapy (ergotherapy) – philosophy, objectives and methodology. Rehabilitation Medicine and the Quality of Life. 2007; (2):16 [In Bulgarian].
15. Hansen RA, Atchison B. Conditions in Occupational Therapy. – Baltimore: Williams & Wilkins. 1993; 38-43; 112-134.
16. Hiraoka K. Rehabilitation effort to improve upper extremity function in post-stroke patients: A meta-analysis. Journal of Physical Therapy Science. 2001; (13):5-9.
17. Ivanov V, Takov E, Tivchev P. Fractures – diagnosis and treatment. – Sofia: Venel. Tom 2, 1996; 196-215 [In Bulgarian].

18. Kalchev I, Morova E. Kinesiology. – Sofia: University "Sv. Kliment Ohridski". 1993; 45-52; 107-129 [In Bulgarian].
19. Kapandji IA. The physiology of the joints. – London: Livingstone. 1970; 72-79.
20. Kaplan E, Tzurengapova D, Shantanova L. Optimization of the adaptive processes of the organism. – Moskow: Science. 1990; 137-149.
21. Kaptelin LF, Lasskay LA. Occupational therapy in traumatology and orthopedics. – Moscow: Medicine. 1979; 91-93; 131-132 [In Russian].
22. Karaneshev G, Milcheva D. Methods for diagnostics and examination in remedial gymnastics. – Sofia: National Sport Academy. 1984; 26-73 [In Bulgarian].
23. Karaneshev G, Sokolov B, Venova L et al. Edited by G. Karaneshev. Theoty ang methods of remedial gymnastics. – Sofia: Medicine and Physical Culture. 1983; 62-69; 97-103; 149-152; 188-201; 217-223; 261-262 [In Bulgarian].
24. Katirji B, Koontz D. Disorders of peripheral nerves. In: Daroff RB, Fenichel GM, Jankovic J, Mazziotta JC, eds. Bradley's Neurology in Clinical Practice, 6-th ed. – Philadelphia, Pa: Saunders Elsevier. 2012; 76-82; 114-119.
25. Kielhofner GA. Model of Human Occupation. – Baltimore: Williams & Wilkins. 1995; 80-93.
26. Kojuharov V. Kinesiology analysis of the gripping power of the hand with fingers reconstructed. Proceedings of II Congress of the Association of Kinesitherapeutists Rehabilitators and Bulgaria. Sofia, 1989; 13-15 [In Bulgarian].
27. Koleva I. Physical analgesia in neurological diseases. Cephalgia. 2006; 8(1):10-21 [In Bulgarian].
28. Koleva I. Capabilities of modern physical and rehabilitation medicine to improve the quality of life patients. Rehabilitation medicine and quality of life. 2007; 1(1):4-13 [In Bulgarian].
29. Koleva I. Professional competence of bachelors in Medical Rehabilitation and Ergotherapy, as members of the rehabilitation team. Prevention and rehabilitation. 2008; 2(1): 2-7 [In Bulgaria].
30. Koleva I. The bulgarian neurorehabilitation school and the international classification of functioning, disability and health (icf): integrating icf requirements into clinical practice. J. Biomed. Clin. Res. 2009; 2(1):8-18 [In Bulgarian].
31. Kostadinov D, Gacheva Y, Tsvetanova L. Manual Physical Therapy. – Sofia: Medicine and Physical Culture. Tom 1, 1989; 64-67; 103-106 [In Bulgerian].
32. Krakauer JW. Motor learning: Its relevance to stroke recovery and neurorehabilitation. Current Opinion in Neurology. 2006; (19):84-90.
33. Krug G. Occupational Therapy: Evidence-Based Interventions for Stroke. Missouri Medicine. 2009; (106:2):145-149.
34. Latham NK, Jette DU, Coster W et al. Occupational therapy activities and intervention techniques for clients with stroke in six rehabilitation hospitals. American Journal of Occupational Therapy. 2006; 60(4):369-378.
35. Legg LA, Drummond AE, Langhorne P. Occupational therapy for patients with

problems in activities of daily living after stroke. Cochrane Database of Systematic Reviews. 2006; (4):583-585.

36. Logan PA, Gladman JRF, Avery A, Walker MF, Dyas J, Groom L. Randomised Controlled Trial of an Occupational Therapy Intervention to Increase Outdoor Mobility after Stroke. BMJ. 2004; (25):1136-1139.

37. Matev I, Bankov St. Rehabilitation of Hand Inguries. – Sofia: Medicine and Physical Culture. 1977; 32-38; 67-75; 79-84; 121-135 [In Bulgarian].

38. Matev I. Reconstructive surgery of the thumb. – Sofia: Medicine and Physical Culture. 1978, 14-25. In Bulgarian].

39. Mihaylova N. Occupational Therapy in some degenerative diseases of the motor support apparatus. – In: Topuzov I, editor. Occupational Therapy: II part. – Sofia: RIK Simel. 2008; 68-76; 153-155 [In Bulgarian].

40. Ministry of Education, Bulgaria. Ordinance on Unified State Requirements for Obtaining Higher Education in professional field of "Health Care" educational and qualification degree "specialist". Published by the Official Gazette, number 95/ 29.11.2005 [In Bulgarian].

41. Ministry of Health – Programme Phare. Health reform in Bulgaria. Collection of lectures, first part. Floor. order. Prof. M. Popov. – Sofia: Makedonia press. 1997; 382 [In Bulgarian].

42. Mok E and Woo CP. Slow stroke massage helps stroke patients. Complementary Therapy Nurse Midwifery. 2004; (4):209-216.

43. Mollova K, Paskaleva R. Rehabilitation activities in patients with motor dosturbancer. Collection materials of International cientific conferention – Stara Zagora's bads. 2009; 32-35 [In Bulgarian].

44. Morov Sp. Human Anatomy. – Sofia: Medicine and Physical Culture. 1981; 68-91; 154-179 [In Bulgarian].

45. Nabi A. The innovative work of the teacher in the system of quality assurance. Problems of modern Philology, Pedagogics and Pshichology. Materials digest of the XXV International Scientific and Practical Conference in Pedagogics, Pshichological sciences and the Philological sciences. Pedagogical Sciences. – London. 2012; 17-19 [In Russian].

46. Ovcharov Vl. Morphology of pain. – B: Pain – pathogenesis and treatment. Edited by P. Shotekov. – Sofia: Leader press. 1998; 146-149 [In Bulgarian].

47. Orjeshkovskiy VV, Volkov ES, Gabrikov NA et all. Klinicheskaya physiotherapy. – Kiev: Health. 1984; 393-395 [In Bulgarian].

48. Paskaleva R. Kinesitherapy motivating role in the fight against obesity. Prevention and Rehabilitation. 2011; (1):23-29 [In Bulgarian].

49. Paci M. Physiotherapy based on the Bobath concept for adults with post-stroke hemiplegia; A review of effectiveness studies. Journal of Rehabilitation Medicine. 2003; (35):2-7.

50. Pedreti LW, Early MB. Occupational therapy – Practice Skills for Physical Disfunction. Fifth Edition. – USA: St. Louis – Mosby – Elsevier. 2005; 345-367.
51. Petkova I. Interactive methods in educators' qualification, Qualy educayion for all through improving teacher training. Paradigma. 2010; 214-216 [In Bulgarian].
52. Petkova I. Interactive methods in the qualification of professionals working in institutions. Collection of materials International cientific conferention "Interactive methods in modern education" West University „Neofit Rilski". – Blagoevgrad: Sani – H and H OOD. 2010; 368-373 [In Bulgarian].
53. Popov N, Dimitrova E. Kinesitherapy in orthopedic diseases and injuries of the upper limb. – Sofia: NSA – Press. 2007; 295-323 [In Bulgarian].
54. Punwar AJ. Occupational Therapy. – Baltimore: Williams & Wilkins. 1994; 269-273.
55. Reed K, Sandarson S. Conceps of Occupational therapy. – USA – Lippincott: W & M. 2004; 384-391.
56. Regan WD, Korinek SL, Morrey BF ann KN. Biomechanical Study of igaments around the Elbow Joint. Clin. Orthop. 1991; 170-179.
57. Rockwood and Masten. The Shoulder. – Philadelphia: W.B. Saunders Company. 1998; 2 ed.; 1316-1323.
58. Rusk H. Rehabilitation Medicine. – St. Louis, 1964; 38-49.
59. Schleenbaker RE, Mainous AG. Electromyographic biofeedback for neuromuscular reeducation in the hemiplegic stroke patient: A meta-analysis. Archives of Physical Medicine and Rehabilitation. 1993; 74(2):1301-1304.
60. Sinaki M. Basic clinical rehabilitation medicine. – Toronto – Philadelphia: W. B. Saunders Co. 1987; 42-51.
61. Sinelnikov R. Atlas of Human Anatomy. – Moskow: Medicine. 1978; 261-272 [In Russian].
62. Slanchev P, Bonev L, Bankov St. Textbook on Kinesitherapy. – Sofia: Medicine and Physical Culture. 1986; 25-52; 103-106; 119-123; 146-147; 152-154; 246-247; 268-269 [In Bulgarian].
63. Shiflett S, Nayak S, Bid C et al. The effect of reiki treatments on functional recovery in patients in poststroke rehabilitation: a pilot study. The Journal of Alternative and Complementary Medicine. Mary Ann Liebert. 2002; 8(6):755-763.
64. Shy ME. Peripheral neuropathies. In: Goldman L, Schafer AI, eds. Cecil Medicine, 24-th ed. – Philadelphia, Pa: Saunders Elsevier. 2011; 428-431.
65. Steultjens EMJ, Dekker J, Bouter LM, Van de Ness JCM, Cup EHC, Van den Ende CHM. Occupational Therapy for stroke patients: A systematic review. Stroke. 2003; (34):676-687.
66. Solgard S, Petersen VS. Epidemiology of distal radius fractures. Acta Orthop Scand. 1985; (56):391-393.
67. Stucki G, Ewert T, Cieza A. Value and application of the ICF in rehabilitation medicine. Disability and Rehabilitation. 2002; (24):932-938.

68. Swanson AB, Matev I, G. de Groot. The strength of the hand. Bulletin of Prosthetics Research. 1970; 145-153.
69. Takov E, Tivchev P, Ivanov V. The fractures – diagnostic and treatment. – Sofia: Venel. II part, 1996; 127-135; 305-328 [In Bulgarian].
70. Ternovoy KS, Kravchenko AA, Leshtinskiy AF. Rehabilitation Therapy in Trauma Locomotory System. – Kiev: Health. 1982; 65-71; 103-111 [In Russian].
71. Titynova E. Brain reorganization after a stroke. Neurorehabilitation. 2008; 2(2):22-26 [In Bulgarian].
72. Topuzov I. Occupational Therapy. – Sofia: RIK Simel. II part, 2008; 101-109 [In Bulgarian].
73. Topuzov I. Occupational Therapy. – Sofia: RIK Simel, III part, 2009; 73-79; 213-224 [In Bulgarian].
74. Trombly CA. Occupational Therapy for Physical Dysfunction. – Boston – Baltimor – Philadelphia – Hong-Kong – London – New York – Sydney – Tokyo: Williams & Wilkins. 1996; 121-127; 216-232.
75. Tsairis P, Dyck PJ, Mulder DW. Natural history of brachial plexus neuropathy. Report on 99 patients. Arch Neurol. 1972; (27):109–117.
76. Vacheva D, Mircheva A. Complex functional assessment of recovery for injuries and diseases of the upper limb. International Scientific Conference "Modern methods and technologies in research" – Proceedings of the University of Economics – Varna. 2012; 420-462.
77. Vacheva D, Simeonova V, Stamenov B. The Recovery Detection of Daily and Labor Activities in the Everyday Life in Patients who Suffered from Cerebral Vascular Disease. Acta Med. Bulg. 2013; XL(2):46-52.
78. Vasilievoy V. Therapeutic Physical Culture. – Moscow: Medicine. 1970; 119-127 [In Russian].
79. Walker MF, Gladman JRF, Lincoln NB, Siemonsma P, Whiteley T. A randomised con-trolled trial of occupational therapy for stroke patients not admitted to hospital. Lancet 1999; (354):278-280.
80. World Health Organization. International Classification of Functioning. Disability and Health (ICF), WHO, Geneva, 2001.
81. Yates DW. Trauma – British medical bulletin. 1999; 55(4):181-186.
82. Yiancheva S, Milanov I, Georgiev D, Shotekov P. Motor activity. In: Yiancheva S, editor. Neurology – General neurology. – Stara Zagora: College. 1998; 105-109; 204-227 [In Bulgarian].
83. http://www.aafp.org/afp/2000/1101/p2067.html
84. http://www.advancedreconstruction.com/brachial-plexus-injuries
85. http://emedicine.medscape.com/article/1175276-overview

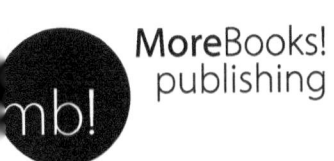

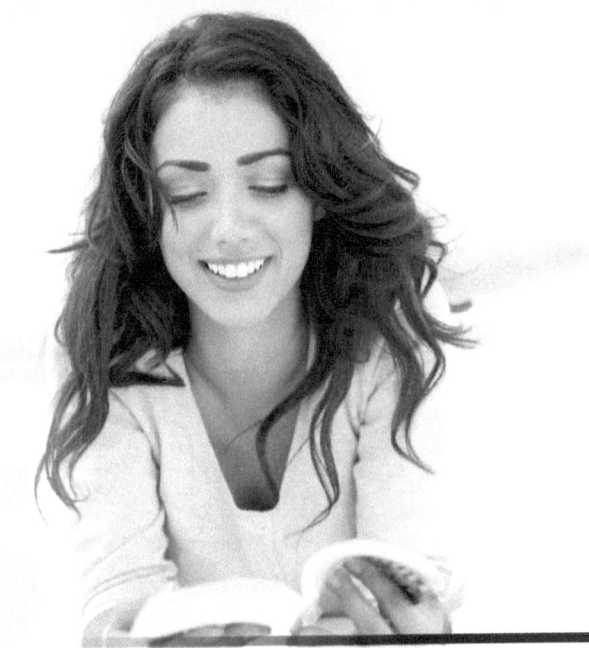

i want morebooks!

Buy your books fast and straightforward online - at one of world's fastest growing online book stores! Environmentally sound due to Print-on-Demand technologies.

Buy your books online at

www.get-morebooks.com

Kaufen Sie Ihre Bücher schnell und unkompliziert online – auf einer der am schnellsten wachsenden Buchhandelsplattformen weltweit! Dank Print-On-Demand umwelt- und ressourcenschonend produziert.

Bücher schneller online kaufen

www.morebooks.de

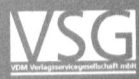

VDM Verlagsservicegesellschaft mbH
Heinrich-Böcking-Str. 6-8   Telefon: +49 681 3720 174   info@vdm-vsg.de
D - 66121 Saarbrücken   Telefax: +49 681 3720 1749   www.vdm-vsg.de

www.ingramcontent.com/pod-product-compliance
Lightning Source LLC
Chambersburg PA
CBHW031547210526
45464CB00003B/1195